Philip Henry Pye-Smith

Syllabus of a Course of Lectures on Physiology

Philip Henry Pye-Smith

Syllabus of a Course of Lectures on Physiology

ISBN/EAN: 9783337173517

Printed in Europe, USA, Canada, Australia, Japan

Cover: Foto ©ninafisch / pixelio.de

More available books at **www.hansebooks.com**

SYLLABUS

OF A COURSE OF

LECTURES ON PHYSIOLOGY

DELIVERED AT GUY'S HOSPITAL.

BY

P. H. PYE-SMITH, B.A., M.D., F.R.C.P.,

Physician to the Hospital.

WITH DIAGRAMS

AND

AN APPENDIX OF NOTES AND TABLES.

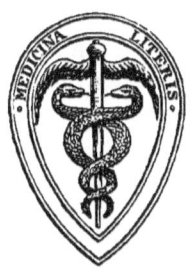

LONDON:
J. & A. CHURCHILL,
11 NEW BURLINGTON STREET.
1885.

PREFACE.

The following pages are the outlines of lectures given at Guy's Hospital during the last ten years, with additions which each year has made necessary. The Diagrams and the Tables in the Appendix are also part of what have been used in the same Course.

In following the example of the late Dr. Alfred Swayne Taylor —one of the best lecturers I ever heard—at Guy's, and of Dr. Burdon Sanderson at University College, I have endeavoured to make the syllabus useful to students, as a help in their systematic reading and self-examination; and also to those who have passed the earlier stages of studentship, in recalling the more important outlines of the "Institutes of Medicine." I have also, I trust successfully, endeavoured to make it useless to any one who may try, "for the purpose of examination," to substitute hasty and ill-digested reading for slowly and practically acquired knowledge.

In case any fellow-lecturer on Physiology should glance at these pages, I may perhaps add that increasing experience in teaching has led me to diminish every year the number of facts taught, and to spend more and more time in the full explanation and repeated statement of those which are most essential.

Results of analysis, and other numerical statements, are best given in tables hung up to be copied. Most experiments are best performed by, or in presence of, a limited number of students in laboratory classes, such as I have held every summer session. But in every course of lectures on physiology there should find place some few fundamental experiments— such as demonstration of digestive processes, of Blood-pressure and the action of the Heart, of the nervous regulation of the Circulation and Respiration, and of the simpler functions of Muscle and Nerve. Easily seen demonstrations of a few of the most important physical and chemical properties of the organs are also extremely useful. But these all need to be carefully led up to and fully explained. Lastly, I would urge the value of rough, and if possible, home-made models or "tangible diagrams" of the structure of muscle and nerve fibres, of blood-disks, of the ovum and embryo, of the eye and internal ear, of the course of fibres in the brain and cord, of the mechanism of the thorax, and of the circulation—from a leaden tube to an elaborate "schema."

On the principle of fulness rather than multiplicity, I have been in the habit of prefacing the account of each group of organs by a brief notice of their development and comparative anatomy, and also of admitting some historical details into the exposition of such fundamental doctrines as the Conservation of Energy, the Coagulation of the Blood, the Circulation, Oxydation and Respiration, Secretion, Animal Temperature, and Embryology. By exhibiting the works and, when possible, the portraits of eminent physiologists, and by reading original passages from such authors as Harvey, Mayow, Hales, Bichat, Magendie, Marshall Hall, Johannes Müller, Bernard, Ludwig, or Helmholtz, personal interest may be given to dry discussions; and the results of science will be all the better understood if the process by which they were reached is, however imperfectly, followed.

I have been reminded of intelligent and responsive audiences and of valued laboratory assistants, while writing out these pages. They may perhaps serve to recall not unwelcome memories to some of those who have now become my fellow-students in the still wider and more engrossing field of Medicine.

HARLEY STREET,
December, 1884.

CONTENTS.

SYLLABUS OF LECTURES.

	PAGE
Introductory: Definitions—Relations of Physiology to other Sciences and to Medicine—Methods	1
General Construction of the Body	5
Its Chemical Constituents	7
Its Physiological Elements and their Functions	12
A. Nutrition—Food—Digestion	19
Absorption and Bloodmaking	22
Circulation of the Blood	25
Respiration—the Voice	29
Excretion and Secretion	33
Review of Nutritive Changes—Balance of Material	38
B. The Work of the Body—Balance of Energy—Temperature	41
The Nervous System	43
The Special Senses	48
C. Reproduction and Development	55

APPENDIX.

1. The term "Physiology"	61
2. Classification of the Sciences	62
3. Characters of the Organic Kingdom	64
4. Distinctive Characters of Animals and Plants	64
5. Anatomical Characters Peculiar to Man	65
6. Definitions of Disease	66
7. Observations and Experiments upon Oneself	67
8. The Conservation of Energy	68
9. The Branchial Arches, Clefts and Nerves	69
10. Table of the Bones with their Homologues	70
11. Table of the Chemical Elements of the Body	73
12. Table of the Proximate Principles of the Body	74

CONTENTS.

	PAGE
13. Table of the Reactions of the Principal Carbohydrates	76
14. Pflüger's Table	77
15. Physical Laws affecting Absorption	78
16. Comparison of Lymph, Chyle and Blood	78
17. Physical Laws affecting the Circulation	79
18. Table of Events in a Cardiac Cycle	80
19. Statistics of the Circulation	81
20. Physical Laws affecting Respiration	82
21. Statistics of Respiration	82
22. Table of the English Vowels	83
23. Table of the Consonants	84
24. Comparative Wasting of the Organs in Starvation	86
25. The Material Balance of the Body in Health	86
26. Table of the Relative Energy available from various Foodstuffs	87
27. The Balance of Energy	87
28. Outgoings of Energy in the Form of Heat	88
29. Table of Temperatures	89
30. The Centres and Commissures of the Nervous System	90
31. Physical Properties of Light	91
32. Physical Properties of Sound	91
33. Varieties of Segmentation	92
34. Chronology of the Chick in the Egg	93
35. Chronology of the Fœtus in Utero	95
36. General Statistics of the Human Body. Total weight—Proportions of Water, of Salts, of Fat—Weight of Organs	96
37. Table of British Weights and Measures	99
38. Table of Centigrade Weights and Measures	100
39. Relations of British and Centigrade Tables	100
40. Relations of Fahrenheit and Centigrade Scales	103
41. Lists of Important Names and Dates in the History of Physiology : viz.	
I. Of Anatomy	104
II. Of Histology	105
III. Of Physiological Chemistry	106
IV. Of the Progress in Knowledge of the Nutritive Functions	107
V. Of the Functions of the Nervous System	108
VI. Of Development	109

LIST OF DIAGRAMS.

I. The Digestive Apparatus.
II. Incomings and Outgoings during Digestion.
III. Absorption.
IV. The Systemic Circulation.
V. The Nerve-Centres which regulate the Circulation.
VI. The Principal Nerves which regulate the Circulation.
VII. The Apparatus of Respiration.
VIII. The Respiratory Mechanism of the Thorax.
IX. The Respiratory System of Nerves.
X. The Vocal Apparatus.
XI. The Mechanism of Secretion.
XII. Nervous Regulation of Secretion.
XIII. The Balance of Material.
XIV. The Balance of Energy.
XV. The Elementary Nervous Combinations.
XVI. The Projection System.

SYLLABUS

OF

LECTURES ON PHYSIOLOGY.

INTRODUCTORY.

PHYSIOLOGY: "The Science of the Functions of Living Creatures" (see *Note* 1 in Appendix for the origin and use of the word).

Science: Knowledge; exact knowledge; measurable knowledge. Natural Science. Natural History and Civil History. Natural History and Natural Philosophy. "Descriptive" and "Rational" Sciences. Observation and experiment. Facts and events. Sequence of events. Causal relation of events.

Classification of the Natural Sciences (see *Note* 2 in Appendix). Comte's; Spencer's; relation of Physiology to Anatomy (structure and function), to Chemistry and Physics (physical and vital actions).

Function: action; movement; duty; use.

The utility of "organs" or instruments; what each does; how it does it; how organs and functions have been reciprocally developed.

Living beings: Life, a popular, not a scientific term; ambiguous; "the condition of organized creatures," or, "the supposed cause of this condition." Living things

B

organized; organisms; distinctive characters of organic and inorganic bodies (see *Table* in Appendix, No. 3).

Human Physiology: its relation to general Biology, to Vegetable and "Comparative" Animal Physiology; distinctive characters of animal and vegetable organisms (see *Table* 4). Distinctions between man and lower animals (*Note* 5).

Normal Physiology: its relation to pathology or morbid physiology; Health and Disease, popular, not scientific, terms. (*Note* 6).

General Human Physiology: its relation to the actual physiology (and pathology) of each individual; to the physiology of sex; of infancy, youth and age; of race and occupation. The ideal physiological man.

Material Physiology: its relation to Psychology. Consciousness; body and mind; limitation of physiology as a natural science.

THE STUDY OF THE BODILY FUNCTIONS OF HEALTHY HUMAN BEINGS.

Relation of Physiology to Medicine: the Institutes of Medicine. Pathology, or the study of the bodily functions under injury or disturbance. A corresponding knowledge of the functions under the action of drugs and other remedies would make a complete scientific basis for the practice of medicine.

Methods of Physiology: Observation and experiment—*i.e.*, observation under purposely varied conditions.

Direct observation—*e.g.*, of movements of glottis in speech by laryngoscope; of stomach during digestion, by a fistula; of mammalian heart exposed during artificial respiration; of muscle of frog after removal from body.

Experiments upon man or animals by varying food, exercise, temperature, &c.—*e.g.*, excretion of urea. Accidental experiments made on man by injury or by disease. Designed experiments on the lower animals involving injury. Importance of direct experiments on man when practicable and harmless (*Note* 7). Difficulties of interpreting the experiments made by disease. So-called vivisection; its necessity and justification; its safeguards and limits.

Life and Vital Force: Mutual dependence of structure and function. *E.g.*, movement performed by a muscle; muscular tissue produced by growth, nutrition, differentiation. Power of growth and movement dependent on the properties of protoplasm; this derived from preceding living parent. *Omne vivum ex ovo;* seeds and eggs; equivocal generation; Redi; modern experiments.

Origin of living protoplasm and of vital functions as unknown (and probably unknowable) as the origin (or mode of creation) of matter and of force.

"Explaining" phenomena means referring them to already known causes.

In this sense *vital force* is now explained. It is the chemical force of attraction which keeps together the elements of food. This latent energy becomes kinetic under suitable stimuli, in the forms of mechanical movement (of muscles, cilia, &c.) and of heat (vital warmth); with less important transformations into electro-motive energy (*e.g.*, *Gymnotus*) or radiant light (*e.g.*, *Noctiluca*).

Correlation of forces; conservation of energy (*Note* 8).

Animals derive their "vital force" from plants: plants theirs from the rays of the sun; chlorophyll; fixation of carbon. Animals expend the stored energy of food in movement. Plants also expend energy in growth, reproduction, and, to a limited extent, in heat and in motion, *e.g.*, cilia, *Mimosa pudica*, slow geotropic movements; but their chief function is storing food and energy, making starch from carbonic dioxide and water, and converting kinetic solar energy into latent chemical energy.

Hence the chemical differences between animals and plants; the leaves and roots of the one kingdom, the stomachs of the other; and the presence of special instruments of movement in animals alone. (See *Table* 4.)

In both kingdoms the living functions may be grouped as follows :—

1. *Nutritive,* including growth, assimilation, decay, and death.

2. *Reproductive:* formation of buds, ova, sperm-cell; fertilization, and detachment of the new organism.

. *Functions of relation* by which the organism is acted on by surrounding objects and reacts upon them. Irritability; manifested in sensation and in movement.

The two former kinds of activity are as much developed in plants as in animals, and may therefore be called " vegetative ;" the last is distinctively (though not exclusively) "animal." The first and last are for the maintenance of the individual; the second is for the maintenance of the race. The first is storing of matter and of energy; the latter two are the expending functions.

THE GENERAL CONSTRUCTION OF THE BODY.

All animal and vegetable structures made of cells and their products.

Cell (corpuscle, plastid)—original meaning; the vegetable vesicle of Grew, the cell of Schleiden, the animal cell of Schwann: "cell-wall, cell-contents, nucleus;" solid cells, naked cells. *Protoplasm* (Von Mohl, Reichert, Max Schultze), structureless, granular, reticulated; albuminous, with water and salts, particularly phosphates; power of growth, nutrition, irritability, movement, reproduction.

Def. Cell : a minute mass of nucleated living protoplasm.

Origin of all the tissues from the germ-cell or ovum; the morula or mass of segmentation cells; the hollow blastoderm; its three layers, upper, lower, and mid-most, called epi-, hypo-, and meso-blast, or ecto-, endo-, and meso-derm.

Comparison of this development of the organism from the ovum (Ontogeny) with the evolution of the more complex from the simplest organisms (Phylogeny).

The uni-cellular Protozoa. Colonies; mouth; *Gastræa;* blastopore; differentiation from one into two layers (endo- and ecto-derm) by *dilamination,* by *invagination;* formation of body cavity (*cœlom*) and mesoderm in Cœlenterata; formation of anus. Elongated form; sense organs; head; movement; bilateral symmetry. Segmentation; somites; serial symmetry, in worms, insects, vertebrates. Limbs in symmetrical pairs, limited to two pairs in Vertebrata; tail, a swimming organ; legs, wings, and hands. Dorsal position of nervous system in Vertebrata. Fore, mid, and hind gut; primitive symmetry of stomach, liver, heart; vascular arches with branchial clefts, and aorta (*Note* 9). Nephridia, Wolffian bodies and kidneys.

Homology of the vertebrate skeleton.

Centra; neural arches; visceral or body-arches; central axis; neural and oral arches of skull; splint bones; hyoid and branchial skeleton.

Limbs: shoulder-girdle and pelvis; distal segments.

(See Table of Bones with their Homologues. *Note* 10.)

THE CHEMICAL CONSTITUTION OF THE BODY.

ELEMENTS.—Organic Chemistry, the chemistry of Carbon compounds; combining powers of carbon. All food which supplies energy consists of carbon-compounds; all living stuff or protoplasm of nitrogenous carbon-compounds; hence the four most abundant and important elements of the animal body are *Carbon* and *Nitrogen*, with *Oxygen* and *Hydrogen*.

Sulphur and *Phosphorus*: partly associated with them in living tissues, partly forming metallic sulphates and phosphates.

Chlorine and *Fluorine*, forming salts with metals. These metals all alkaline—viz., *Sodium* and *Potassium*, *Calcium* and *Magnesium*.

Lastly, *Iron*, found only in hæmoglobin and its derivatives. (See *Table* 11.)

PROXIMATE PRINCIPLES.—A. Inorganic, mineral: water and salts. B. Organic, non-nitrogenous: carbohydrates and fatty compounds. C. Organic, nitrogenous: proteids and crystalline bodies (*Table* 12).

I. WATER.—More than two-thirds of the whole weight, about three-fourths of the soft tissues, four-fifths and upwards of the liquids, and only about one-tenth of the skeleton. Unchanged chemically in its passage through the body. Its solvent and diffusive power; relation to heat; necessity to the colloid condition.

II. SALTS.—Soda salts characteristic of animal, as potash of vegetable, tissues; NaCl more abundant in the liquids, K and phosphates more abundant in the tissues than the liquids, earthy salts more abundant in the hard parts.

$NaCl$; Na_3PO_4; Na_2HPO_4; NaH_2PO_4; Na_2SO_4; Na_2CO_3; with corresponding salts of K.

$Ca_3 2PO_4$; $CaCO_3$; CaF_2, with corresponding salts of Mg.

None changed in passage through body except from acid to neutral or alkaline or the reverse.

Mechanical function in the bones and teeth; solvent and diffusive power of crystalline salts and of alkalies in the liquids; constant and probably essential presence of salts, especially phosphates, in protoplasm.

III. CARBOHYDRATES: $C_m(H_2O)_n$. — Connection through mannite with the group of polyatomic alcohols, aldehydes and ethers. Gum, lignin and cellulose, starch (granulose), and sugars (*Table* 13). Importance in food; scanty and transitional presence in products of digestion and in the tissues: cellulose in Tunicata; starch granules in green Hydra; diabetic sugar (Willis, 1660); animal starch or glycogen (Claude Bernard, 1860).

Glycogen, $C_6H_{10}O_5$: properties, mode of preparation, presence in liver, muscles, blood, leucocytes, placenta, and fœtal tissues generally.

Glycose, $C_6H_{12}O_6$, and *maltose*, $C_{12}H_{22}O_{11}$, products of digestion of starchy food; present in traces in normal blood and probably in urine.

Lactose, $C_{12}H_{22}O_{11}$, presence in milk.

Inosit, $C_6H_{12}O_6$ (Scherer), in muscles of heart and elsewhere.

IV. HYDROCARBONS.—Less oxidized than starches; inflammable; high degree of latent energy. Fats solid, and oils liquid, at ordinary temperatures. Animal and vegetable oils. All glycerides of fatty acids; one, two, or three of the movable H-atoms in the triatomic alcohol, propyl-glycerine $\overline{C_3H_5}'''(OH)_3$ being replaced by the radical of a fatty acid (Chevreuil, Berthelot). The fats of the human body (beside traces of glycerides of other fatty acids, as butyric and caproic in milk and sebum): tripalmitin, tristearin, triolein; compounds of glycerine with the 16th and 18th of the acetic or "fatty" acid series ($C_{16}H_{32}O_2$ and $C_{18}H_{36}O_2$), and with the 18th of the acrylic acid series ($C_8H_{34}O_2$).

Refracting power; colour; relation to water, alcohol, ether; fusibility, saponification. Occur, in the proportion palmitin, stearin, olein, in the cells of adipose tissue and yellow marrow, and of the liver; in chyle, in blood, in the secretions of the mammary and sebaceous glands; and, in combination with phosphoric acid and neurin, as *lecithin* in the brain, nerves, bile, and blood corpuscles.

V. PROTEIDS, or albuminous group: Comp. C above half by weight, H about 7 per cent., O about 21, S ·5 to 1·5, N the remainder; constantly associated with water and with salts, some portion of which (especially of the phosphates) is inseparable; colloid (crystalline forms; of vegetable proteids, as aleurone-granules, of albumen (?) in minute hexagonal crystals, of hæmoglobin), non-diffusible (except peptones); soluble in water, or saline, or alkaline solutions; insoluble in alcohol and ether.

The three proteid colour tests: *xanthoproteic* with HNO_3 and a caustic alkali, violet with *copper*, mulberry pink with *Millon's* mercurial reagent.

Decomposition into CO_2 and H_2O, and ammoniacal compounds as leucin, tyrosin, aspartic and glutamic acids; existence in a soluble and a coagulable form; lævogyrate; insoluble compounds with tannic acid and salts of mercury and other heavy metals.

Albumins. Soluble in distilled water: coagulable at 70° C.: also by strong mineral acids and by picric, tannic, and nascent ferrocyanic acid. Varieties in serum, "serum-albumins," coagulating at two or three points; in bird's eggs, "ovalbumin," and in vegetable tissues.

Globulins. Soluble in saline solutions; coagulable at various temperatures; precipitated by weak acids, as acetic, and by CO_2, and also by saturation with neutral salts. The nearest approach to the chemical composition of living protoplasm in cells. Varieties: *crystallin*, from the lens; *paraglobulin* from serum; *fibrinogen* from plasma; *fibrin*; *myosin* from muscle; *vitellin* from yelk.

Alkali-albumin. Derived from all albumins or globulins; native in milk (casein) and in pulse (legumin); absent from blood. *Acid-albumin* a corresponding product with acids.

Peptones. Digested albumins, globulins, acid or alkali albumins; most soluble, least readily precipitated, and least indiffusible of the proteid group.

VI. OTHER COLLOID NITROGENOUS COMPOUNDS DIFFERING MORE OR LESS FROM TRUE PROTEIDS.

Mucin. Soluble in alkaline solutions; imperfect proteid reactions; yields leucin and tyrosin.

Gelatin. Soluble in warm water; insoluble compounds with tannic acid and perchloride of mercury; larger percentage of N; yields leucin and glycin.

Chondrin. Soluble in warm water, precipitated by acetic acid; intermediate between mucin and gelatin.

Elastin. Its great power of resisting solvent and decomposing agents.

Keratin. Its large percentage of sulphur.

Lardacein, pyin, and other pathological products.

HÆMOGLOBIN. Crystalline though non-diffusible; its spectrum; its condition as oxidized and reduced; its natural products, *hæmatoidin, bilirubin* and the yellow pigments; its artificial products, *hæmatin* and globin, *hæmin,* &c.

CRYSTALLINE NITROGENOUS COMPOUNDS. — Chemical composition ascertained; simpler derivatives of the albuminous group; excreta.

Taurin (amido-isethionic acid) and *glycin* (amido-acetic acid) combined with cholic acid and sodium in bile.

Leucin (amido-caproic acid) and *tyrosin* (oxyphenyl-amido-propionic acid) found in the urine in disease.

Urea (carbamide) the chief solid constituent of the urine.

Creatin (rational formula unknown, hydrated creatinin) in muscle-extract, and *creatinin* ($C_4H_7N_3O$) in urine.

Uric Acid ($C_5H_4N_4O_3$) in urine, free in disease, normally as a soda salt. *Xanthin* ($C_5H_4N_4O_2$), occasionally present in urine. *Hypoxanthin* ($C_5H_4N_4O$) in muscle extract.

Cystin (amido-sulpholactic acid), occasionally present as urinary calculus.

Hippuric acid (benzoyl-glycin; constantly present in

combination with K and Na in the urine of men, and more abundant in that of purely vegetable feeders.

Indol (C_8H_7N) occurs in the intestine, and *indican* occasionally, blue *indigo* very rarely, in the urine.

Sulphocyanide of potassium (KCNS) is always present in the saliva.

THE PHYSIOLOGICAL ELEMENTS OF THE BODY AND THEIR FUNCTIONS.

Elementary tissues: Classification by Bichat, by Virchow.

FREE CELLS, like uni-cellular protozoa, in animal liquids: *Leucocytes, Blood-disks, Ova, Spermatozoa.* Comparison of leucocytes to amœbæ, of ova to encysted, and of sperm-cells to flagellate, Infusoria.

CELLS CONJOINED IN COLONIES—EPITHELIA. Classification:
a. In one layer or several.
b. The component cells: Size. Shape: spheroidal (polyhedral), long (prismatic, cylindrical or columnar, conical, &c.), flat (squamous, tessellated, or pavement epithelium). Edges: hexagonal, wavy, serrated or cogwheel, or "prickle-cells." Nucleus: shape, size, situation; absent in old epithelium. Protoplasmic network and rods. Vacuoles: granules, oil-drops; "signet-cells." Cilia.
c. Chemical characters: Globulin, crystallin, keratin, mucin, earthy salts, pigment.
d. Origin: From epi-, hypo-, or meso-blast.
e. Functions: Protective, diminishing friction, absorbent, motor, refractive, secreting.
f. Pathology.

Practical recognition of three principal orders of epithelium:—

(1) Epithelium (*sensu restricto*).
(2) Epidermis.
(3) Endothelium; intercellular "cement."

Resemblance between (1) and (2); relation of (3) to the following group.

THE PHYSIOLOGICAL ELEMENTS OF THE BODY. 13

CONNECTIVE TISSUES: Cells with an intercellular matrix or ground-substance; all meso-blastic.

a. Fibrous tissues: Cells fusiform, stellate, flat and oblong, winged, globular and vacuolated; matrix of white or yellow fibres.
Varieties:
White fibrous and yellow *elastic* tissue mingled in different proportions and arranged in wavy bundles, parallel lines, and laminæ, felted or reticular. Relation to lymphatic spaces and to endothelium. *Areolar*, or connective tissue proper.
Adipose tissue, with large signet-cells filled with oil: fat and yellow marrow.
Corneal tissue.
Neuroglia.
Gelatinous (myxomatous or œdematous fœtal) connective tissue.
Retiform (lymphatic or cytogenic) tissue.

b. Cartilage: Cells oval, in alveoli, loculi, lacunæ or capsules of the matrix; matrix various; yields chondrin.
Varieties:
Embryonic or cellular; scanty matrix.
Hyaline or alveolar; granular or glassy matrix.
White fibro-cartilage; few cells.
Yellow elastic or reticular fibro-cartilage; felted matrix.

c. Calcified:
Varieties:
Bone: cells oval, stellate; matrix fibrous, petrified. Peculiar arrangement in Haversian systems; where nutrition is from periosteum, this arrangement absent and why.
Dentine or ivory: cells in pulp cavity with processes in dentine tubules; intercellular matrix.

Note.—Connection of these apparently dissimilar tissues; in essential structure, in chemical products (gelatin, chondrin, and mucin), in derivation from mesoblast, in functions (chiefly mechanical with important exceptions in adipose and cytogenic tissues), in pathology; substituted one for the other in development, in comparative anatomy, and in disease and repair.

Higher tissues : more differentiated ; the constituent cells no longer obvious ; muscle and nerve.

MUSCLE : consists of fibres, with nuclei representing cells ; yields myosin ; has the power of contraction carried to perfection.

Varieties :

Unstriated or "smooth," or "involuntary" muscular fibre ; narrow, flattened, pale nucleated fibres, and constituent fusiform muscle-cells ; slow contraction.

β. Cardiac fibres : Imperfectly striated, anastomosing, broad fibres, resolvable into short, oblong, nucleated muscle-cells.

γ. Striated, striped or "voluntary" fibres. Size $\frac{1}{2}$ by $\frac{1}{400}$ inch. Transverse, alternate dim and bright striæ, sarcolemma, nuclei, sarcous elements (or muscle prisms, or muscle rods), united by interstitial cement into fibrillæ (elements in file) and disks (elements in rank) ; Goodfellow's and Dobie's dark line (Krause's so-called membrane) dividing bright striæ ; its interpretation. Appearance with polarized light, singly (aniso-tropic), and doubly (iso-tropic) refracting parts ; effect of reagents ; appearances during contraction and stretching ; cause of the striation.

Fibres bound together by connective tissue (endomysium) into bundles (fasciculi), these surrounded by more connective (perimysium), which separates the fasciculi (septa), and invests the whole muscle (fibrous sheath or fascia propria). Bloodvessels, with oblong meshes, and saccular dilatations ; lymphatics, nerves, interstitial fat, form, with the white and yellow connective fibres, the stroma of a muscle.

Tendons : Structure ; connection with muscular fibres and with bone.

Physical properties of living muscle at rest : transparent ; red with a pigment identical with, or closely allied to, hæmoglobin ; elastic (very distensible, and recovers almost perfectly ; curve of elasticity) ; alkaline ; "natural" electrical current.

Chemical constituents : water ; salts, especially K & P ; pigment (hæmoglobin), glycogen, myosin ; muscle-plasma.

Muscular contraction: not coagulation of myosin or "inogen;" comparable to amœboid, ciliary and flagellate motion. Phenomena of contraction: the blood-vessels dilate; each fibre becomes shorter and broader; bulk not changed; more distensible; small amount of heat evolved; negative variation of current of rest; chemical changes; CO_2 produced (even in N); reaction becomes acid, $C_3H_6O_3$; alcoholic extractives increased; bruit musculaire.

Method of registering a muscular contraction; the muscle-curve; time of each part; latent period; double stimulation. Tetanus; its curve.

Effects of resistance, as raising a weight, on contraction. The source of muscular energy; means of measuring the work done; degree of contraction in frog's muscle, in human. Length, the measure of possible range; cross-section or number of fibres, of possible strength.

Effect of contraction on hollow cavities (bladder, heart), or cylinders (intestine, bronchus, artery), or openings (iris, pylorus); effect where both ends are movable (arytænoideus); when either is movable (hamstrings); when one only is movable (facial muscles, masseter); change of direction of pull in trochlear muscles (superior oblique, obturator internus); composition of forces in penniform and bipenniform muscles, and in muscles with a common insertion (quadriceps, iliaco-psoas).

Muscles always on the stretch, not only from elasticity, but also from slight reflex contraction ("tonus"); use of muscles as elastic ligaments, capable of tightening when required.

Contraction of unstriated muscle; of red and pale striated muscles in the rabbit.

Death of muscle: Coagulation of myosin; rigor mortis; its rapidity and duration; how distinguished from a true contraction.

NERVE.—Consists of ultimate fibres of protoplasm with or without sheaths; function, to conduct stimuli.

Varieties: a. Fibres with double contour; medullated or

white fibres. Continuous axis (or axis-cylinder) of fibrillated protoplasm, surrounded by white sheath of myelin yielding ordinary fats, lecithin, cholesterin, &c., and by an external structureless "primitive sheath," the neurilemma; nodes of Ranvier, how demonstrated; nuclei; comparison of each node with a muscle-fibre-cell.

β. Non-medullated grey fibres of Remak; axis cylinder with nuclei and neurilemma, but no myelin investment; proportion to white fibres in olfactory nerves, in sympathetic branches, in optic, and in spinal nerves.

Fibres bound together by connective tissue (endoneurium) into bundles (funiculi), these united together in large nerve-trunks by perineurium, which invests the whole as a remarkably strong fibrous sheath (formerly called "neurilemma"). Scanty blood-vessels.

Chemical constituents: Water, salts (especially phosphates), fatty matter, protagon, lecithin, cholesterin, and globulin.

Physical properties of living nerve: Transparent, single contoured (the myelin being uncoagulated) with a "natural nerve current." When active—*i.e.*, conducting—the current suffers negative variation; with slight thermal and chemical changes (?).

Effect on conductivity and irritability of moderate and gradual heat and cold, of moisture and dryness, of exhaustion, and of the passage of a weak continuous galvanic current (electrotonus; an- and cat-electrotonus, neutral point).

Stimuli to nerve (beside the physiological stimuli): mechanical from end-organs or ganglia; thermal; chemical (not identical with those of muscle); electrical (especially the induced current; different effects of a descending or ascending current, of making or breaking the current, of strength of the current; Pflüger's table and his law thence deduced (*Table* 14). Greater effect of the momentary induced (or faradic) current over the make or break of a primary (or galvanic) current.

Rate of nerve conduction in motor nerves; in afferent; in frog, mammalia, man; influence of fatigue, &c.

Nature of nerve-current unknown; physical or chemical. Proof that it is not an electric current.

Afferent or centripetal; efferent or centrifugal; and commissural or intercentral nerve fibres. Direction of current probably determined by terminal connection (comparison with telegraph wires).

Peripheral terminations of nerve fibres : (1) In free extremities or anastomosing loops or plexuses, after the axis cylinder has lost its medullary sheath and neurilemma, and has broken up into its constituent fibrilla—cornea, skin, between the epithelial cells.

(2) In motor end-plates in striated muscle; Doyère's description in Tardigrade Crustacea, Kühne's in lizards; also in mammals.

(3) In Pacinian bodies (Vater, Pacini, Herbet) : in the digital nerves, mesentery, corpora cavernosa, &c.; and in tendons, tongue, &c.

(4) In corpuscula tactûs (Meissner), in end-bulbs (Krause) and their modifications: in the cutaneous papillæ, the conjunctiva, the mucosa of the genital organs, in joints, and in the tongue and beak of birds.

(5) In end-organs of modified epithelium, as the rods and cones of the retina, the hair-cells of the cornea, &c.

(6) In the secreting epithelium of glands.

(7) In the electrical organs of the torpedo and gymnotus.

GANGLIA consist of a group of large nucleated cells with processes, connected with each other and with nerve-fibres, and imbedded in a ground substance of neuroglia.

Ganglion cells or nerve corpuscles—size, shape, stellate, pyriform, oval, &c.; peculiarities in the anterior cornua of the cord, the cerebellar cortex, the ganglia of the posterior nerve-roots, the several regions of the cerebral cortex, &c. Always with two processes at least. Nucleus, nucleolus, granules, sheath.

Connection with nerve-fibres by an (unbranched) axis-cylinder process.

Function : reception of stimuli from afferent and origination of stimuli to efferent nerves. Power of storing stimuli. Spontaneous or *automatic* and reflected or *reflex* " explosions " of ganglion cells.

Stimuli to ganglia, probably the same physical excitants as those of muscle and nerve, but during life either an afferent nerve-current (reflex) or chemical change in the afferent blood (automatic), or (by an inscrutable connection) the mental condition called Will (conscious automatic activity).

Irritability of ganglia increased by heat, lowered by cold, increased by strychnia and diminished by morphia.

Combination of afferent and efferent nerve and ganglion into a reflex system. (Diagr. XV. A.)

Combination of ganglion with ganglion to check its action—Inhibition. (Diagr. XV. F.)

FUNCTIONS OF NUTRITION.

These include: the Prehension, Digestion, and Absorption of food; its conversion into Blood; the distribution of this liquid food to the tissues by the mechanism of the Circulation; the Growth of the tissues; their Oxydation, with the Excretion of the resultant products: the subsidiary processes of Secretion by which solvent juices and waste products are separated from the lymph; and lastly the Nervous mechanisms which regulate and control the above processes.

The study of the processes of decay and death of the tissues, and of the organism, is part of the physiology of Nutrition; but is for convenience relegated to the department of Morbid Physiology (Pathology) or the science of the functions in disease.

Food.

Inorganic food of plants absorbed from outside by the leaves or roots—Carbon from the air, Water from the soil, and Nitrogen, with Salts in solution, from the soil. Power of decomposing CO_2 under sunlight by the parts containing chlorophyll or leaf-green.

Food of Animals. Organic compounds, with water and salts.

Uses: (1) to provide and maintain the elements of the tissues, *i.e.*, water and salts (Na, K, Ca, Mg and Fe, with Chlorides, Phosphates, Sulphates, and a trace of fluorides), the Carbon characteristic of all organic compounds, and the Nitrogen characteristic of active and especially of animal tissues.

(2) to provide energy in the form of oxydisable (*i.e.*, combustible) compounds of C and H with or without N.

(3) to stimulate nerves and glands.

GROUPS OF FOODSTUFFS.

Inorganic. { I.—Water
            { II.—Mineral Salts { Soluble. / Insoluble. } } Incombustible.

Non-Nitro Organic. { III.—Carbohydrates { Starches. / Sugars. }
                   { IV.—Fats
                   { V.—Nitrogenous: (1) Proteids.
                       (2) Gelatin, &c. } Combustible.

The first of the above objects is fulfilled by I., II., and V., which are therefore called *tissue-forming*; the second by III., IV., or V., which are mutually replaceable; the third by minute quantities of food, chiefly nitrogenous, which appear to act as drugs, by stimulating to sensation and secretion. These may be called " Adjuvants," and include :

(1) Relishes—*e.g.*, the savoury constituents of meat.
(2) Condiments—*e.g.*, salt, spices, &c.
(3) Stimulants—*e.g.*, wine, tea, &c.

Result of deprivation of water—of salts—of all non-nitrogenous organic matter—of either oily or starchy food—of osmazome and other " extractives " of meat.

Effects of cooking—*i.e.*, either dry heat, or heat and moisture, or starch : on fats : on albumin, myosin, globulin, hæmoglobin : on connective tissue and gelatin.

Prehension: of solids; of liquids, drinking.

DIGESTION.

The chemical process of rendering food soluble and more and less diffusible. No digestion of water and salts, which pass through the body unchanged, except in the case of salts of vegetable acids, which are excreted as carbonates.

Comminution, preparatory to solution.

Gizzards. Stomach-teeth : splanchno-skeleton : tooth-like structures in epiderm of certain vertebrates.

TEETH.—Calcification of mucous membrane covering the jaws (præmaxillary—maxillary—mandibular, palatal, pterygoid, and pharyngeal teeth): *enamel* or calcified epithelium; *dentine* (ivory) or calcified corium; pulp or uncalcified

I. DIAGRAM OF THE DIGESTIVE APPARATUS.

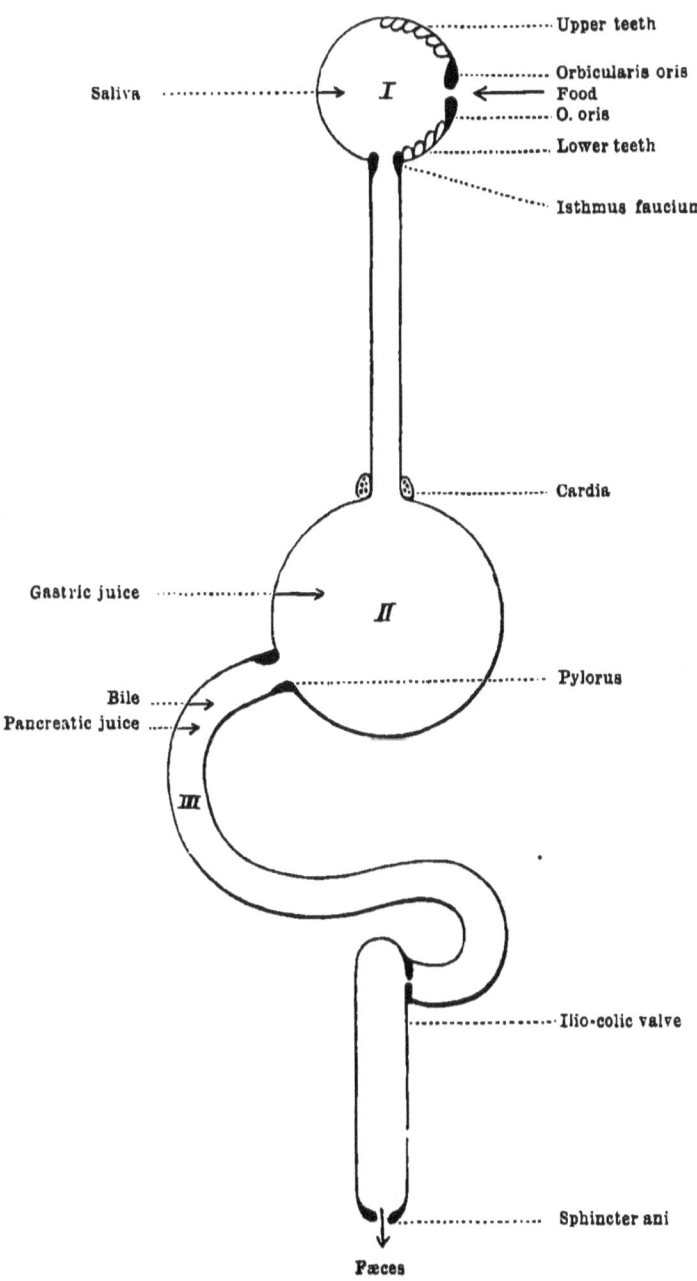

To face page 20.

Passage of food through pylorus. Regurgitation. Rumination. Vomiting. Post-mortem digestion of the stomach itself.

PANCREATIC DIGESTION. Pancreatic secretion. Reaction, ferments.

Stages of digestion. Proteids, alkali-albumin, Peptone. Part of this unchanged ("Anti-peptone"), the rest ("Hemi-peptone") converted into Leucin and Tyrosin. Formation of indol and appearance of bacteria, not essential.

Pancreatic digestion of starch into dextrin and maltose.

Pancreatic digestion of fatty compounds by a ferment ("steapsin") which splits them into the fatty acid and glycerine. Subsequent formation of soap. Small extent of this change during life: its probable significance. Formation of Emulsion by pancreatic juice, independent of a ferment.

RESULT OF DIGESTIVE PROCESSES.—*Chyme.* Water, salts, peptones, and partially digested albuminous compounds, sugar, and fatty emulsion.

The residue, dregs, or *Fæces* : water, insoluble salts, indigestible parts of food, as cellulose and elastin, undigested excess of food as starch-grains and muscle-fibres, residue of ferments, mucus, and constituents of bile.

Large amount of water poured into alimentary canal during digestion and re-absorbed : the vehicle for solution and absorption. Contents less and less liquid in passage through intestine.

Reaction of contents of mouth and œsophagus, alkaline; of stomach acid; of duodenum alkaline; then neutral and fæces usually acid.

ABSORPTION.

Digested food in alimentary canal not " in the body."

Two channels for its conveyance : (1) by the veins of stomach and intestines to the portal vein and liver and thence to the heart; (2) by the lymphatics or absorbents to the thoracic duct and so to the heart.

II. DIAGRAM OF THE INCOMINGS AND OUTGOINGS TO AND FROM THE ALIMENTARY CANAL.

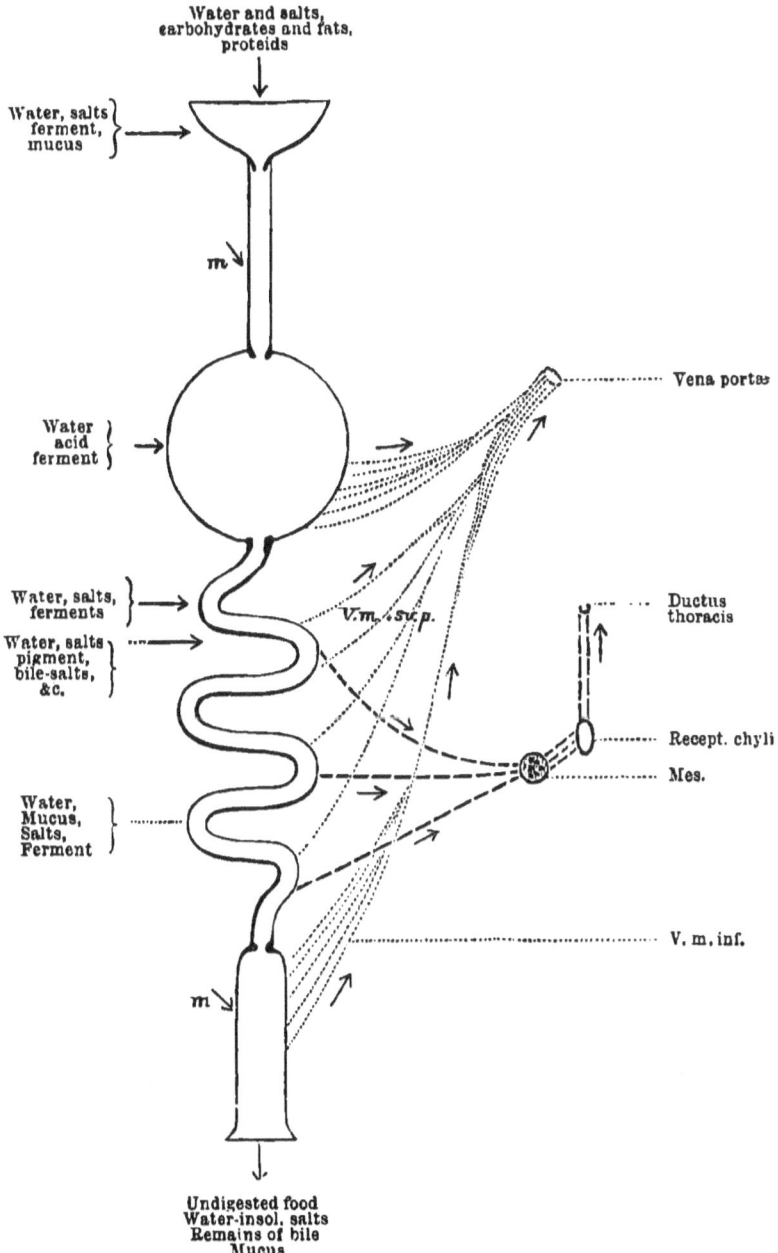

To face page 22.

(c) Elaborated into "lymph-glands" or *lympharia*.

Lymph corpuscles, young leucocytes: white blood-corpuscles, adult leucocytes : inflammatory or granulation corpuscles, out-wandered or emigrated leucocytes: pus-corpuscles, dead leucocytes, undergoing fatty degeneration.

Red corpuscles or blood-disks. Varieties of size and shape among Vertebrata. Absence of nucleus in Mammalia. Origin from leucocytes, in embryo, in adult; not nuclei. Transition-forms in red marrow: qu. also formed in spleen? Change of size and shape, loss of nucleus, loss of contractility. Stroma (œcoid) and hæmoglobin (zooid). Assumption of hæmoglobin.

BLOOD.—Colour. Sp. gr. Reaction. Microscopic characters. Gases. Water. Salines: iron. Aqueous, alcoholic, and etherial "extractives." Proteids.

Coagulation. Not dependent on cooling, rest, or evaporation; nor on exposure to oxygen, or "vitality," or presence of red disks; but on the assumption of the coagulated form by one of the globulin group of proteids. Observations of Hewson, Buchanan, Alex. Schmidt, Hammarsten, and Wooldridge. Action of serum-globulin (paraglobulin or fibrinoplastin) of fibrinogen, of a ferment, of the white corpuscles. Small amount of fibrin formed. Stages of coagulation: viscid condition, solid blood : contracting clot, serum.· Influence of temperature, movement, contact with foreign bodies, dilution. Effect of neutral saline solutions. Coagulation under the microscope. Blood kept liquid by cold ; by preservation in the heart, or in a vein, or in a smooth glass vessel. Coagulation of chyle, lymph, inflammatory exudations, colourless blood of invertebrates.

Practical bearing of the theory of coagulation on ligature of arteries, aneurysm, thrombosis, embolism.

IV. DIAGRAM OF THE SYSTEMIC CIRCULATION.

I. Represents the intrinsic cardiac ganglia
II. The inhibitory ganglia
III. The accelerator ganglia
IV. The vaso-motor centres

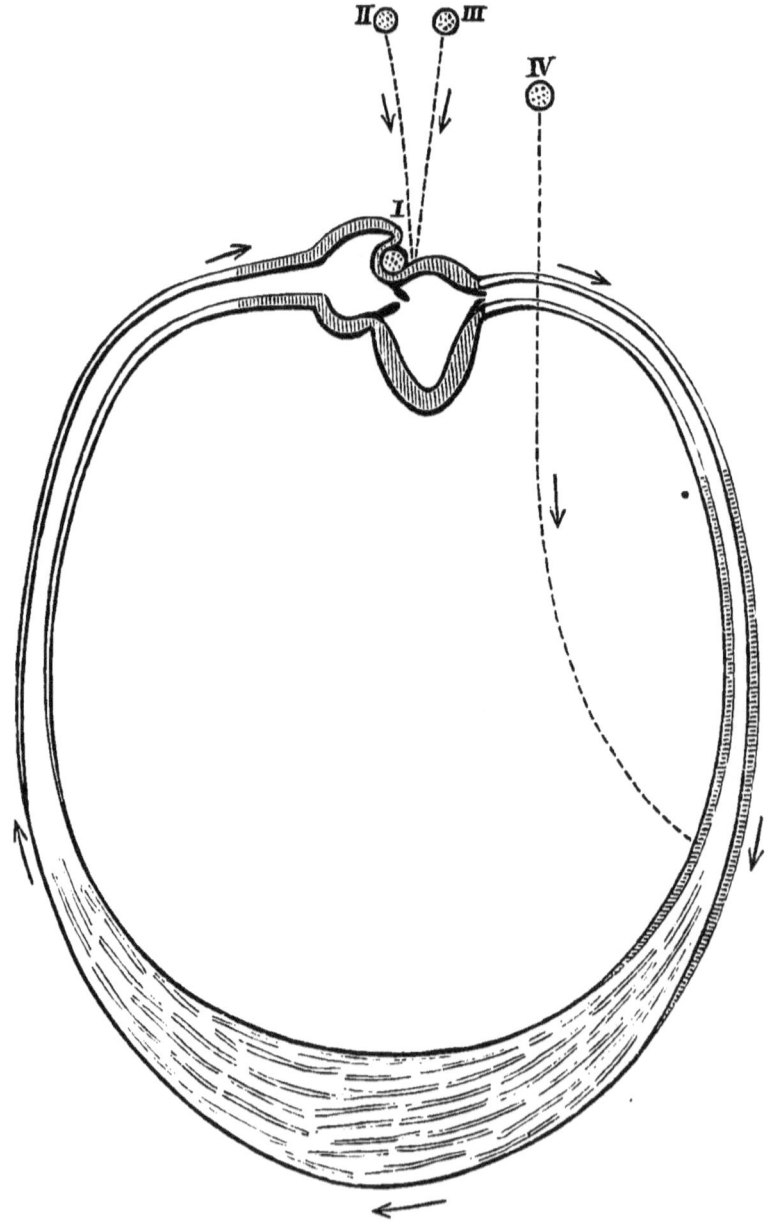

To face page 25.

CIRCULATION.

Functions. Transportation of blood (*i.e.*, of liquid food, water, salts, proteids, sugar and fat) to the living cells of the tissues. Also conveyance of oxygen to tissues, and of waste products thence to excretory organs. Also equalization of temperature.

Apparatus: a closed system of elastic tubes returning into itself. Formed of differentiated mesoblast: endothelial lining, unstriped muscle and white and yellow fibres. Interrupted by a strong contractile chamber, provided with valves of ingress and egress. (Pulmonary circulation postponed.)

Capillaries, permeable, inelastic (contractile). Arteries impermeable, elastic, contractile. Veins less impermeable, less elastic, contractile only in largest trunks and in the great terminal sinus or "atrium" or "auricle." Heart (ventricle) impermeable, elastic, strongly and rapidly contractile.

Hydraulic laws involved (*Table* 17).

Blood pressure: how demonstrated. Hales, Poisseuille, Ludwig, Fick, Landois, Roy. Greatest in ventricle in systole, next in aorta, less in arteries, less in capillaries, still less in veins, lower still in auricle, lowest in ventricle in diastole.

Velocity of blood: how measured. Volkmann, Vierordt, Ludwig, Chauveau. Greatest in aorta, somewhat less in smaller arteries, least in capillaries, more and more rapid as aggregate calibre of veins diminishes.

Pulse: relation to intermittent beat of heart, resistance of small arteries and capillaries, elasticity of aorta and larger arteries.

Blood pressure tracings, sphygmographic tracings. Clinical varieties of pulse.

The efficient forces which carry on the circulation :

(1) Ventricular systole (strength and frequency).

(2) Auxiliary; pressure of muscles during contraction upon the valvular veins; pressure of air in aspiration of thorax; negative pressure in ventricle during systole, owing to its own elasticity.

Function of *muscular coat of arteries* to regulate blood-pressure, to regulate supply of blood to particular organs. Function of *elastic arteries* to store part of the energy of the ventricular systole and pay it back during diastole.

ACTION OF THE HEART. — *Contraction of auricle :* its strength, frequency, duration, relation to ventricular systole. Auricular dilatation and rest.

Contraction of ventricle; not a tetanus; its energy; work done by it, how measured; its frequency (*pulsus frequens aut rarus*) duration (*p. celer aut tardus*) and regularity. It includes (1) preliminary tension or hardening, (2) movement, (3) sustained immobility in systole. *Diastole :* includes dilatation (by elasticity of muscular tissue) and rest or "pause" in dilated state.

Mechanism of valves of egress : obey pressure passively; adaptation of edges; function of sinuses of Valsalva; sudden tension, *second sound*. Aortic obstructive or direct, and leaking or regurgitant murmurs (production of murmurs, "fluid veins"). Mechanism of valve of ingress (mitral): obey pressure passively; mode of shutting; function of chordæ tendineæ and musculi papillares. *First sound :* tension of mitral (and tricuspid) curtains and ventricular walls, with the added bruit musculaire of contraction. Murmurs from narrowing of orifice (direct or obstructive); from leaking of valve (regurgitant), owing to puckering of its curtains, shortening of the chordæ, or want of constriction of the muscular fibres surrounding the orifice.

PULMONARY CIRCULATION.—Essentially like the Systemic. Resistance less; energy less; [orifices rather larger; length

V. DIAGRAM OF THE PRINCIPAL NERVE-CENTRES REGULATING THE CIRCULATION.

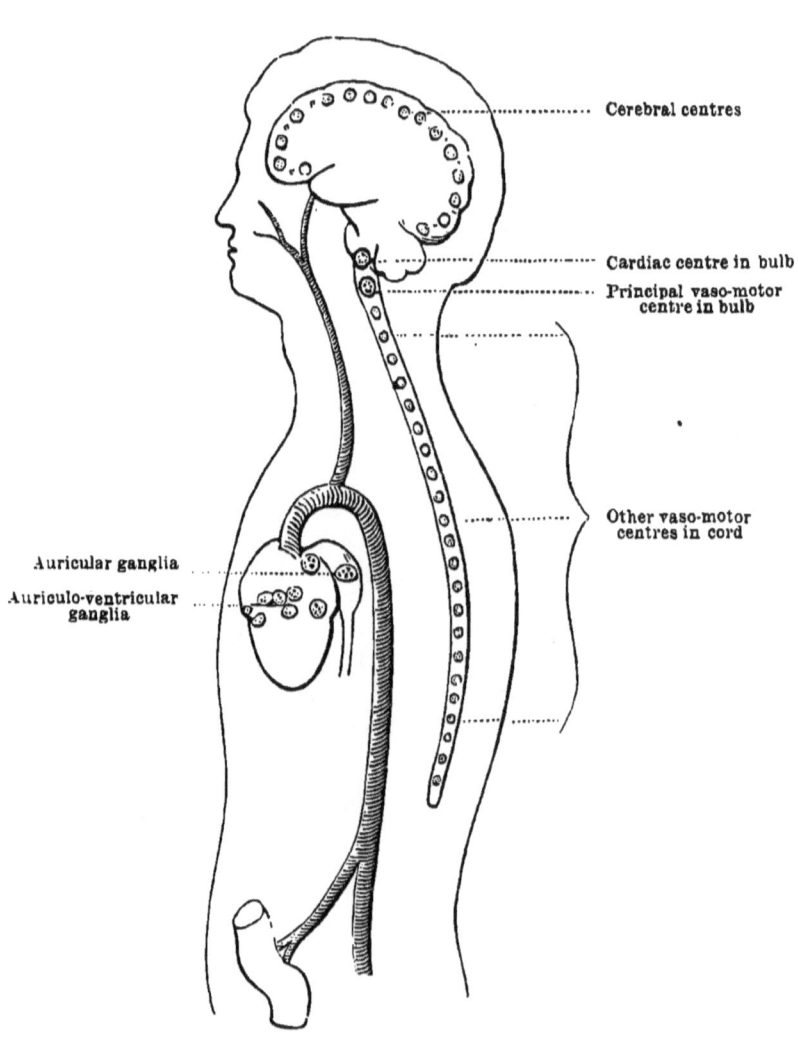

To face page 27.

CIRCULATION.

shorter; friction less;] walls thinner. Blood-pressure lower. Velocity slightly less (?). No auxiliary forces. Systole, diastole, movements of valves, sounds, all synchronous on both sides of heart. Valve of ingress *tri-* not *bicuspid;* consequent safety-valve action; King's " moderator-band; " physiological tricuspid regurgitation.

Change of form of Heart as a whole in systole; apparent elongation; no real locomotion; Cardiac Impulse. Rotation, tilting and hardening of heart. Lengthening and untwisting of aorta and pulmonary artery when distended. " Recoil " from unopposed exit of blood as in a gun or a turbine.

Sequence of events in a complete cycle of the heart's action. (*Table* 18.)

REGULATION OF THE CIRCULATION by the nervous system. Acts only on muscular fibre, (*a*) of heart, (*b*) of arteries.

(*a*) *Cardiac innervation:* in frog: in mammals. Intracardiac ganglia. Rhythmical action: automatic, not reflex. (Exceptional rhythmical contraction of non-ganglionic part of ventricle.) Pulsation of excised heart. Effects of heat, cold, galvanic and faradaic stimulation. Regulation by cerebro-spinal centres. Vagus: inhibitory branches. Stimulation of R. vagus, of L., of both; mechanical, chemical, electrical, reflex: latent period: effect of section of vagi: subsequent effect on beat of vagus-stimulation. Accelerator nerves of heart; section and stimulation of; relation to temperature.

(*b*) *Vaso-motor nerves.*—Cervical sympathetic, splanchnic, brachial, sciatic. Effect on bloodvessels, on the parts supplied, on the blood pressure in front and behind constriction, on B.P. elsewhere, on the pulsation of the heart.

Mutual relation between heart-beat and arterial B.P. and between B.P. and heart. Depressor nerves: other sensory nerves. " Vaso-dilator " nerves. Capillary contraction and dilatation (?).

Effects, on heart-beat and on blood pressure: of dividing Vagi, of stimulating them; dividing accelerator nerves, and stimulating them; dividing cervical sympathetics, dividing splanchnics, and stimulating them; stimulating sensory nerves; destruction of vasomotor centres.

Analysis of tracings obtained from cardiograph (Sanderson), mercurial manometer in carotid (Ludwig), bags in cavities of heart (Chauveau), sphygmograph (Marey).

Statistics of the circulation. (*Table* 19.)

VI. DIAGRAM OF THE PRINCIPAL NERVES WHICH REGULATE THE CIRCULATION.

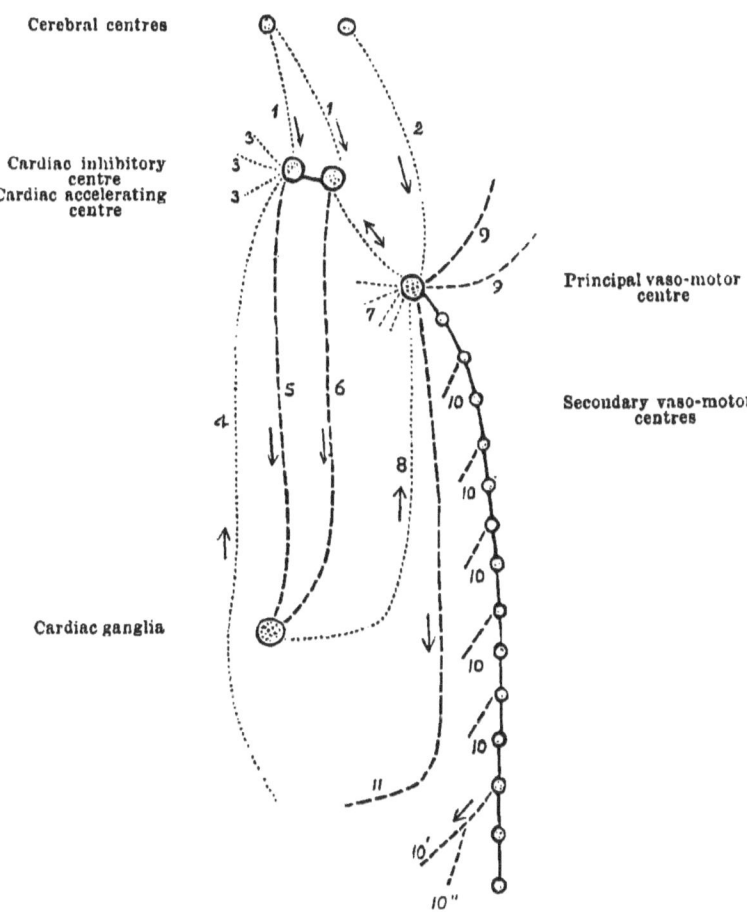

1. Afferent nerves affecting heart by mental emotions.
2.   ,,   ,,   ,,   arteries   ,,   ,,
3.   ,,   ,,   ,,   inhibitory centre from skin of face (5th).
4.   ,,   ,,   ,,   do. from intestines and solar plexus.
5. Inhibitory cardiac fibres of vagus.
6. Accelerator cardiac nerves.
7. Afferent nerves affecting blood pressure through vaso-motor centre in bulb.
8. Depressor branch of vagus from heart.
9. Vaso-motor branches to cerebral, facial, and glandular vessels.
10. Vaso-motor nerves from cord by anterior roots.
10' 10". Separate vaso-motor nerves to vessels of muscles.
11. Splanchnic vaso-motor branches.

To face page 28.

VII. DIAGRAM OF THE APPARATUS OF RESPIRATION.

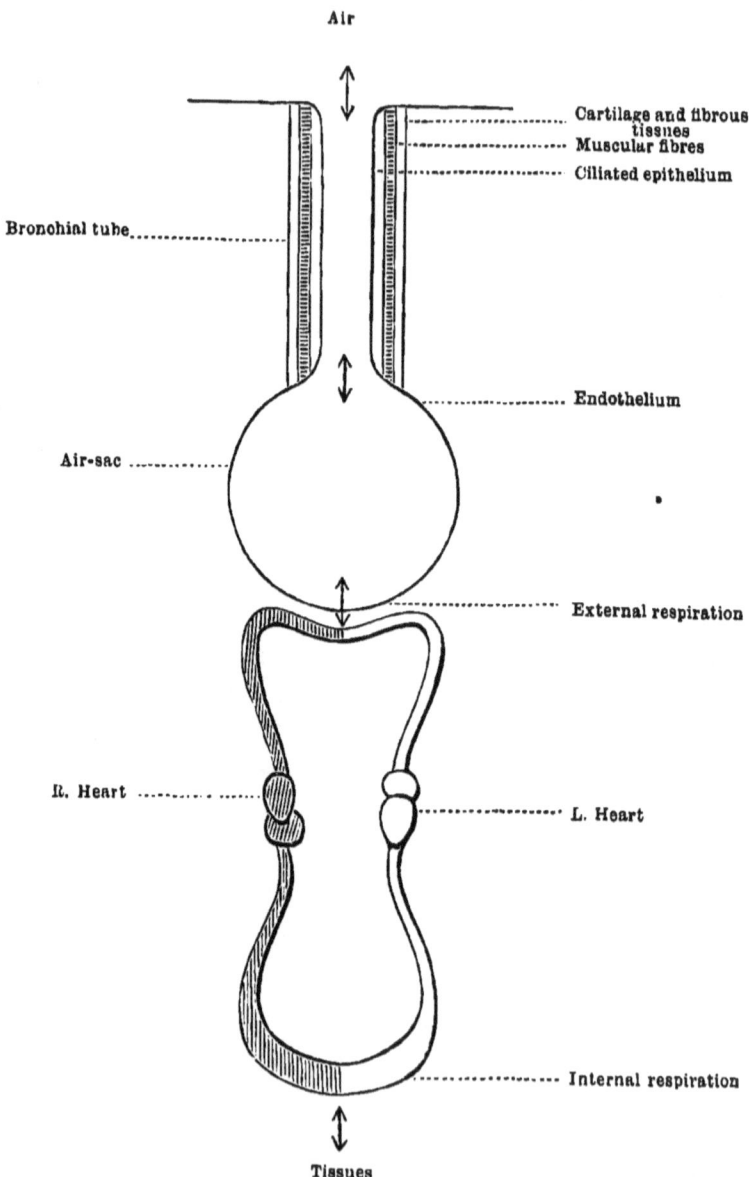

RESPIRATION.

Use made of the liquid food brought to the tissues by the circulation. Need of Oxygen. Chief products CO_2 and H_2O.

Admission of O to the blood from the air, extrusion of CO_2 from the blood to the air, *external* respiration.

Absorption of O from the blood by the living cells, formation of CO_2 and transference to the blood, *internal* or tissue-respiration.

ORGANS OF RESPIRATION. General surface: *skin*. Increased surface by external processes suitable for breathing air dissolved in water : *gills*. Increased surface by internal hollow spaces suitable for breathing air as gas : *tracheæ* bringing air directly to the tissues, *lungs* bringing air to the blood as an intermediary. Outgrowth from gullet : air-bladder and duct in fishes. Lungs of frog, snake, lizard, turtle, birds, and mammals. Nares (not mouth), trachea, bronchi, intra-lobular air-passages, air-sacs (or vesicles or alveoli). Epithelium, cilia. Endothelium, stomata, lymphatics. Elasticity. Vascularity. Muscular fibres of Bronchi. Interlobular connective tissue.

FUNCTIONS. Passage of gases (O and CO_2) between air of alveoli and pulmonary capillaries.

Renewal of air of alveoli from exterior. Physical laws of diffusion and of movement of gases.

Passage of gases between pulmonary vessels and tissues. Solubility in water and serum of CO_2, of O and of N. Hæmoglobin. Oxyhæmoglobin, reduced hæmoglobin. Methæmoglobin. Composition, crystals, colour, spectra. CO_2 conveyed partly in chemical combination.

Renewal of air in lungs. Pneumatic laws involved. (*Note* 20.) Thorax impermeable, resistant and elastic. Expanded in all three directions by muscular effort: inspiration. Diaphragm. Movements of sternum, and of ribs. Contraction by elasticity and by muscular effort: expiration. Action of intercostal muscles. Intra-thoracic pressure. Donders' model.

Changes in air by respiration: O, CO_2, water, nitrogenous putrescible matters: temperature. Changes in blood: colour, O, Co_2, water, temperature in pulmonary capillaries: in systemia.

Statistics of respiration (see *Table* 21).

"Tidal" air of tranquil breathing: "complemental" admitted by extreme inspiration: "reserve" or "supplemental" expelled by extreme expiration: "residual" after such expiration: "post-mortem" air; "tissue" air, of the collapsed lung after opening the thorax. Physical and histological state of a collapsed (airless, carnified) lung, or lobule or lobe.

Frequency and rhythm of respiration. Resp. trace. Inspiratory and expiratory murmur: pulmonary, bronchial, and tracheal sounds. Their conduction to the ear applied to the chest.

REGULATION BY NERVOUS SYSTEM. Respiration automatic, not reflex. Respiration with divided vagi. Stimulation of vagi, of superior laryngeal nerve, of fifth and other cutaneous nerves, of gastric branches of vagus. Expiratory and inspiratory centre in bulb, *nœud vital*: connection with cardiac and vaso-motor centres.

Dyspnœa: from deficient movements of chest: from obstacle to air reaching blood: from obstacle to blood reaching air: from want of hæmoglobin (anæmia): from deficient O in air. Phenomena of dyspnœa and asphyxia.

Apnœa, from excess of oxygen in the blood.

Effect of poisoning by CO_2 in the air: by nitrous oxide, chloroform, ether. Effect of Cl, NH and other irritating gases. Effect of SH_2 and other reducing gases. Effect of CO by

VIII. DIAGRAM OF THE FORCES CONCERNED IN EXPANSION AND CONTRACTION OF THE THORAX.

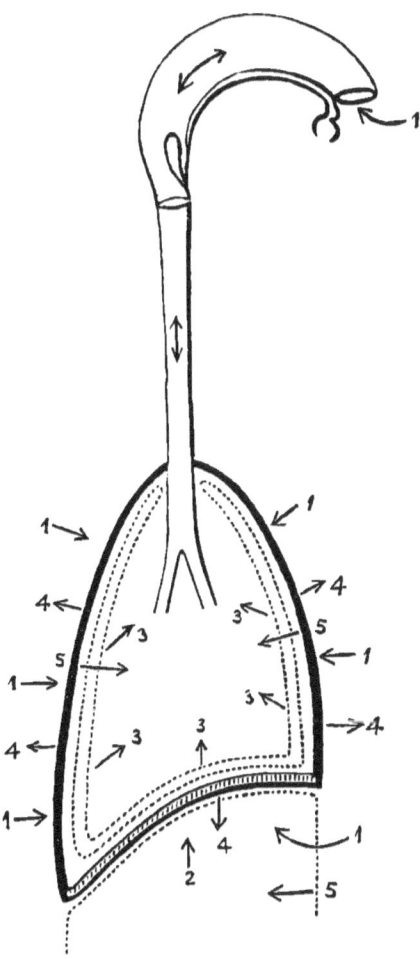

1. Atmospheric pressure on chest, abdomen, and down air passages constant.
2. Upward pressure of abdominal viscera: increased by flatus, ascites, &c.
3. Elastic contractile power of lungs: constant.
4. Expanding power of diaphragm and other inspiratory muscles.
5. Contracting power of expiratory muscles.

The elasticity of the thorax itself comes into action after deep inspiration, and still more after deep expiration.

The double dotted line represents the pleura.

To face page 30

IX. DIAGRAM ILLUSTRATING THE RESPIRATORY SYSTEM OF NERVES.

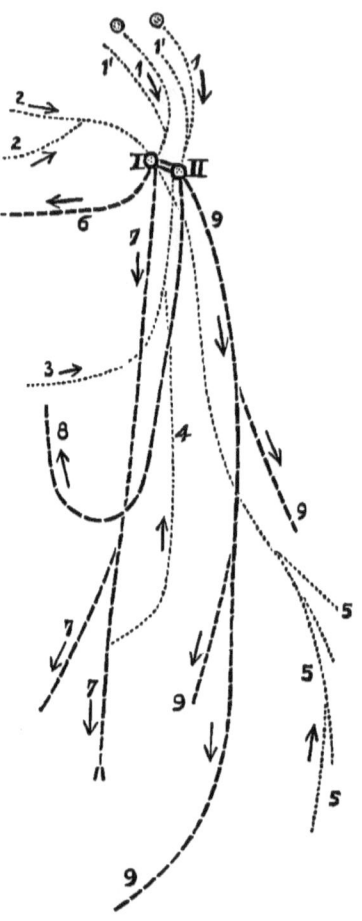

I. & II. Inspiratory and expiratory associated centres in the bulb.
1 1.   Nervous channels for voluntary inspiration and expiration.
1′ 1′. Do. for voluntary inhibition of respiration.
2.   Afferent nerves from retina and skin of face for reflex respiration.
3.   Afferent nerve from larynx.
4.   Afferent fibres of vagus from lungs, stimulant and inhibitory.
5.   Afferent nerves for reflex respiration from skin of trunk.
6.   Motor nerve to dilator of nostrils.
7.   Motor nerves to diaphragm and other inspiratory muscles.
8.   Motor nerves to intrinsic muscles of larynx.
9.   Motor nerves to muscles of expiration.

To face page 31.

its superior affinity to haemoglobin. Effects of air under high and low pressure, suddenly or gradually increased.

Ventilation.

Modifications of the respiratory act: sighing, wheezing, and snoring respiration. Gaping.

Of inspiration: sniffing, gasping, sobbing, hiccough.

Of expiration: sneezing, coughing, blowing, and whistling; gargling; crying and laughing. Vocal expiration.

The Voice.

Its nature. Its qualities:

1. Loudness or amplitude of sonorous vibrations dependent on volume and velocity of expired air. 2. Pitch or rapidity of vibrations, dependent on tension of glottis. 3. "Quality" ("timbre") the presence of overtones or harmonics in addition to the fundamental tone, dependent on the individual structure of the larynx and the "after-pipe."

The mechanism of the voice. Comparable to a reed. Lungs, (bellows) trachea (wind-pipe), glottis ("tongue"), mouth (after-pipe), nose (resonator).

Form of glottis in tranquil and forced inspiration and expiration—respiratory glottis. Form for vocalization—vocal glottis. Muscles opening and closing glottis. Muscles tightening and relaxing cords. Function of ventricle of larynx.

VOWELS: dependent (1) on length of after-pipe; raising glottis and protruding lips; (2) on size of openings of ditto: open or narrow glottis and mouth; (3) on diameter of ditto: raising tongue or depressing floor of mouth; (4) closing resonator: nasal vowels.

Principal and transitional vowels; short and long. Diphthongs. (See *Table 22.*)

CONSONANTS. Expired air stopped more or less completely in after-pipe (1) by lips or incisors, *labials* (2) by tip of tongue and incisors or hard palate, *dentals* (3) by back of tongue and palate, *gutturals*.

Expired air with glottis in vibration, *vocal consonants;* without, *mutes.*

Stoppage incomplete : *continuous consonants, aspirate, sibilant or trilled.* Stoppage complete, *explosives.* Oral stoppage complete with open resonator, *nasals.* Combined consonants. (See *Table* 23.)

Arrangement of alphabet a physiological one. (*Table* 23.)

X. DIAGRAM TO ILLUSTRATE THE VOCAL APPARATUS.

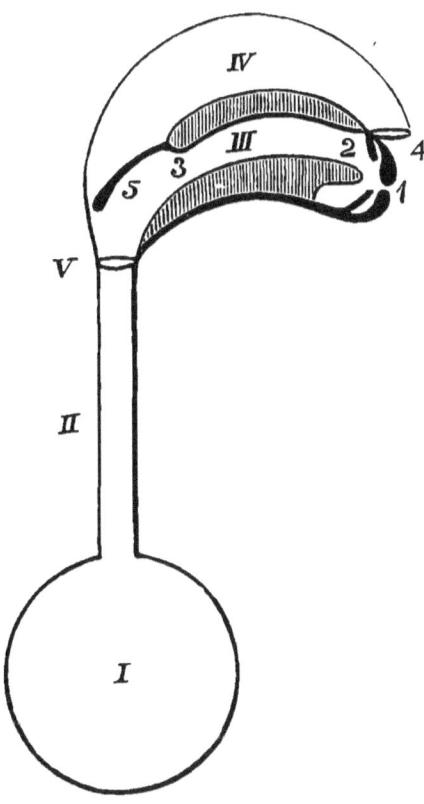

I. Wind-box and bellows.
II. Wind-pipe.
III. Body-pipe.
IV. Resonator.
V. Reed; composed of two vibrating "tongues."

---

1. Anterior consonantal point.
2. Middle do.
3. Posterior do.
4. Anterior opening of resonator.
5. Valve opening or closing resonator.

To face page 32.

XI. DIAGRAM ILLUSTRATING THE MECHANISM OF SECRETION.

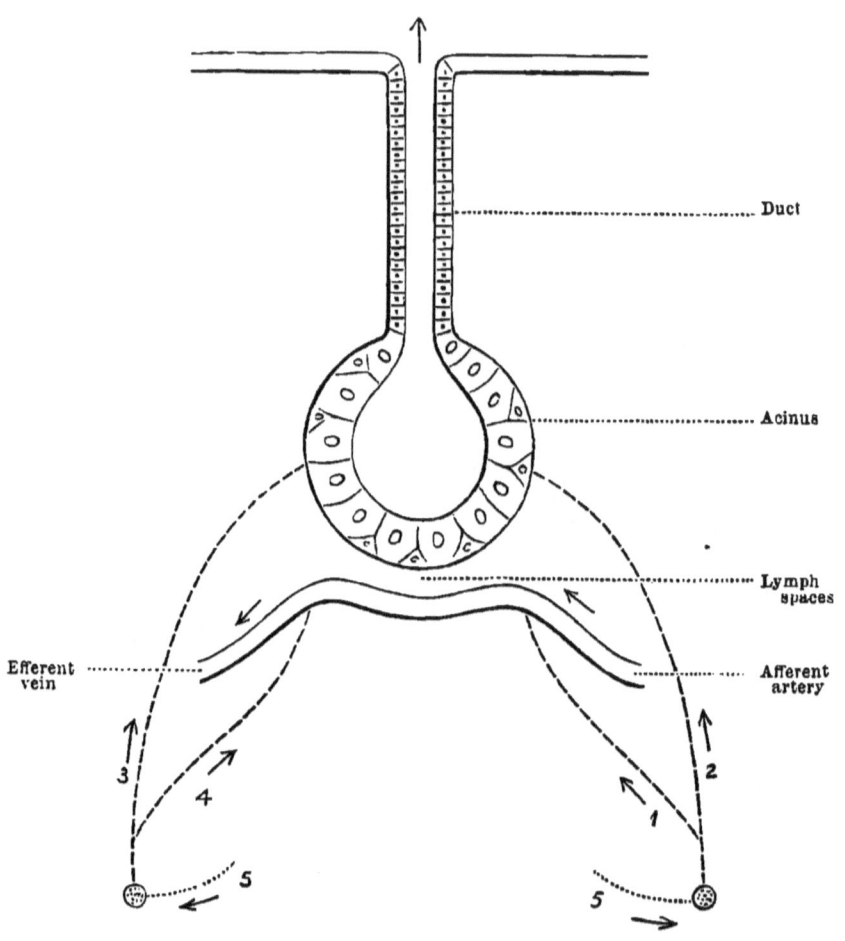

1. Vaso-dilator nerves.
2. Secretory nerves from spinal centre.
3. Secretory nerves from sympathetic.
4. Vaso-constrictor nerves.
5. Afferent, reflex-excitor nerves.

To face page 33.

EXCRETION AND SECRETION.

EXCRETION of waste products. Of C as CO_2, of H as H_2O, of N as urea, of S, P, &c., as salts.

Methods of excretion: by diffusion of gases, by osmosis of liquids, by true secretion.

SECRETION a *process of cell-growth*. Unicellular secreting-glands: goblet-cells. Extension of surface: sacs and pits. Simple saccular depressions—pocketed—more subdivided—racemose—lobulated. Simple deep pits—tubules—branched tubes. Acini and ducts: lobules. Characters of duct-epithelium: of secreting epithelium: transitional forms. Basement membrane. Connective tissue and lymph-spaces. Capillaries. (Diagram XI.)

Regulation by Nervous System. Vaso-motor nerves. Secreting nerves to epithelium of acini. (Diagram XII.)

Secretion as a mere selection of materials ready formed in the blood: as a manufacture of new compounds from those materials.

Process, by transformation of protoplasm of secreting cells; or by vacuolation—"signet-cells." Gradual oozing out of secretion into lumen of acinus; or expulsion by contraction of cell; or liberation by rupture of cell. Comparison of this complete process with storing of secretion, as of starch in roots, and oil in adipose tissue; with ordinary nutrition (every tissue an excretion to every other); with endogenous proliferation.

Histological difference between glands at rest and secreting. "Serous" and "mucous" glands.

Development of glands. i. Glands opening onto skin. ii. Glands opening onto mucous membranes. iii. Genito-urinary glands.

The Skin.

Structure. Epithelium and vascular corium.
Anatomical division.
  i. Epidermis: horny layer or cuticle, Stratum lucidum, S. granulosum, Malpighian layer.
  ii. Cutis vera : papillary layer, deep layer.
  iii. Subcutaneous (adipose) tissue or superficial fascia.
Physiological (and pathological) division.
  i. Dead epidermis, cuticle or scarf-skin.
  ii. Living epidermis and papillary layer.
  iii. Deep layer of cutis and subcutaneous tissue.

Local differences, in the thickness of cuticle, of corium, of integument altogether; in number and size of papillæ; in thickness of subcutaneous layer and in presence of fat-cells; in vascularity; in nervous supply.

Sweat-glands. Structure, number and distribution. Secretion: its composition and reaction. Sensible and insensible perspiration. Effects of temperature, moisture, and movement of the air. Regulation by nervous system. Sweat-nerves, vaso-motor and secreting: warm and cold sweat.

Hairs : structure, distribution and local varieties.

Nails. Structure and use. Formation of nails. Rate of growth. Notches indicative of acute disorders.

Sebaceous glands. Connection with hairs: structure and secretion: function. Modified as Meibomian glands.

Mamma. Collection of highly developed sebaceous glands. Structure in lowest mammalia. Acini, epithelium, ducts, lobules: vessels, lymphatics and nerves. Secretion regulated by N.S. Periodical evolution and involution.

Milk: physical and chemical characters and composition.

Functions of Skin. 1. Protective: nails (hoofs, horny covering of armadillo). 2. Non-conducting: hair (fur), sub-cutaneous fat (blubber). 3. Excretory: of ceratin by abrasion of cuticle and by hair and nails; of water by

XII. DIAGRAM OF THE NERVOUS REGULATION OF SUBMAXILLARY SECRETION.

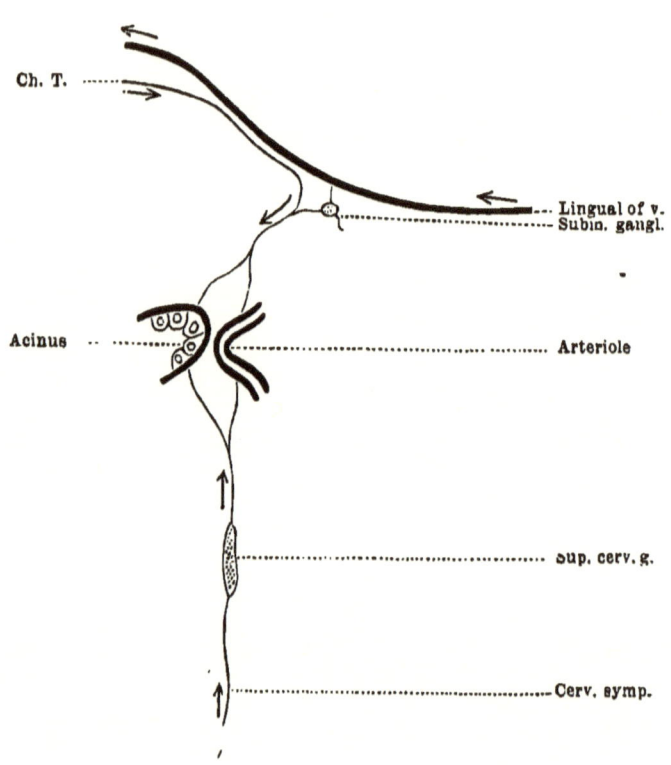

To face page 35.

EXCRETION AND SECRETION. 35

sweat; of sebum. 4. Regulation of temperature (*v. infra*, p. 42). 5. Absorption: not of water, only by inunction.

MUCOUS MEMBRANES AND THEIR GLANDS.

Structure. Epithelium and vascular corium.
 i. One or more layers of epithelium.
 ii. Basement membrane.
 iii. Vascular corium or "mucosa," often cytogenic.
 iv. Submucosa.

Varieties in alimentary canal and in respiratory tract. Mucous glands. Mucus. Succus entericus.

SALIVARY GLANDS. GASTRIC GLANDS. PANCREAS. (*v. supra*, p. 21).

LIVER. Development. Structure. Not racemose nor tubular, nor even properly acinous. So-called lobules unlike those of pancreas or mamma.

Secreting epithelial cells: their structure and arrangement. Variations during digestion: pigment granules, oil-drops, glycogen.

Blood-vessels: Portal interlobular veins and intralobular capillaries ending in intralobular Hepatic vein. Sublobular hepatic veins. Hepatic artery: interlobular and intralobular branches; their termination.

Perivascular connective ("portal canals," Glisson's "capsule") only interlobular and in man very scanty: subserous connective or fibrous tunic.

Ducts: interlobular branches, with mucous membrane; intralobular, an endless network of anastomosing biliary capillaries between the secreting cells: peculiar to the liver.

Lymphatics. Nerves scanty, regulation of secretion by N.S. unascertained.

Bile. Origin of its mucus. Pigments: Bilirubin and Biliverdin. Cholesterin, Lecithin, fats and soaps. Mineral salts. Bile-salts ("bilin" or "bile-resin"): Glyco-cholate and Tauro-cholate of soda (p. 10). *Functions :* not digestive.

Helps to neutralize gastric juice; promotes absorption of a fatty emulsion; antiseptic; stimulates peristalsis and contraction of villi. Water and greater part of conjugated acids reabsorbed. The rest excreted. Peculiarity of secretion: from venous blood, and from blood at low pressure.

Other functions of Liver. Storage of glycogen. Storage of fat. Leuco-cytogenic function in fœtus. Formation of Urea.

KIDNEYS. *Origin* from mesoblast of genito-urinary tract, but in histology and normal and morbid physiology, true epithelium. *Structure* of kidneys. Malpighian capsules and tubules. Endothelium and epithelium. Arteries, glomeruli, venules and venæ rectæ. Connective tissue and lymphatics scanty. Nerves.

Rhythmical contractions as in spleen: relation to general blood pressure. Seat of secretion of water, salts, urea, &c., respectively.

URINE.—An aqueous solution of Urea and NaCl with allied nitrogenous and saline compounds. *Colour.* Concentration; relation of pigment to hæmoglobin. *Sp. gr.* Limits. Relation to food, drink, sweat. Prof. Christison's formula for solids, Dr. Golding Bird's. *Reaction.* Relation to digestion; to vegetable food. Dogs' and rabbits' urine. Dependent on phosphates being acid, or neutral, or basic, with carbonates. *Deposit.* Mucus: whence derived. Epithelium.

Water: amount of urine.

Salts: chlorides, sulphates and phosphates. Occasional presence of carbonates, oxalates, ammoniacal salts, and organic acids, as lactic, succinic.

Urea: composition, solubility and diffusibility. Compounds with Nitric and Oxalic Acids. Mercurial salts. Decomposition into Carbonate of Ammonia by fermentation, into N, CO_2 and H_2O with alkaline hypochlorites or hypobromites. Quantitative tests: Liebig's, the hypobromite,* and complete

---

* Modifications of this process have been brought forward by Leconte, by E. W. Davy (*Phil. Mag.*, June 1854), by Apjohn, Hüfner, Russell and West, and Dupré.

combustion. Relation of urea to muscular exercise: experiments of Fick and Wislicenus, Parkes, Edward Smith, Flint, and Pavy. Relation of urea to nitrogenous food.

Urates of soda and potash. Their solubility dependent on the quantity, alkalinity and temp. of the urine. Their colour. Free uric acid always abnormal. Its physical and chemical properties.

Hippurates constantly present: more abundant in the urine of Herbivora. Preparation, properties and composition of Hippuric Acid. Relation to Benzoic Acid.

Creatinin a nitrogenous crystalline base: its relation to Creatin. Occasional presence of *cystin, xanthin, hypoxanthin* or *creatin* (?) in urine. *Allantoin* in fœtal urine.

Indican: method of testing for.

Gases. CO_2 and N.

Changes in urine after being passed.

Variations by food, temperature, exercise: *Urina somni vel sanguinis, U. cibi, U. potus.* Urine of infant, child, adult. *Morbid urine.*

Mechanism of renal secretion. Arguments from structure and experiments, for the dependence of the watery and saline exosmosis on relative blood pressure in the glomeruli, and of nitrogenous excretion upon the tubular epithelium. Function of looped tubes.

The Bladder: its structure. Mucous, muscular and nervous. Mechanism of micturition.

EXCRETION FROM THE GENITAL ORGANS. *Semen*: proteids and salts of liquor seminis, mucus. Cowper's glands, prostatic glands, vesiculæ seminales. *Ovulation*: menstrual discharge.

REVIEW OF THE FUNCTIONS OF NUTRITION.

Changes of the chemical components of the body, followed from their in-come as food to their excretion. *Metabolism.*

Water, in food, chyme, blood, tissues (see *Table* 36) and excretions.

Salts: slight chemical change from acid to alkali and back, and from citrates, malates, tartrates or acetates to carbonates.

Combustible or oxydizable food stuffs. *Starch and sugars:* conversion into maltose, dextrose, lævulose; reconversion of diffusible crystallines into glycogen; places of origin and storage of glycogen; its further transformation; traces of sugar in the blood; final excretion of carbohydrates as carbonic anhydride and water. Escape of some portion as glycose by the urine in minute traces in health and in quantity in diabetes.

Fats. Absorbed unchanged, in the chyle. Fats in the blood; absence of soaps. Deposit of fat in the liver, and in adipose tissue. Origin of the fat of the body not directly from fatty food; but by indirect process from fat, from carbohydrates (?) and from proteids. Final excretion of fat as carbonic anhydride and water.

Proteids. Absorption as peptones and as particulate albumin. Leucin and tyrosin: relation of both to the fatty acids and of latter to the aromatic series. Serum-albumin and globulin; absence of alkali-albumin in blood. Tissue-proteids: globulin, myosin, gelatin, mucin. Excess of C and H in albumin compared with urea; their detachment in fatty compounds. Lecithin. Conversion of N-residue into crystalline amides and amido-acids. Creatin in muscle and

REVIEW OF THE FUNCTIONS OF NUTRITION. 39

blood ; creatinin in urine. Hypoxanthin, xanthin and uric acid. Glycocholic acid, glycin, tyrosin, benzoyl-glycin or hippuric acid. Taurocholic acid, cystin, sulphates. Antecedents of urea (?), origin in liver (?), absence in muscles, presence in blood, excretion by renal epithelium. Further progress of urea into ammonium carbonate out of the body, or in the inflamed bladder. Hæmoglobin : relation to hæmatoidin, bilirubin and urinary pigment; excretion of Fe. Excretion of proteids as such ; casein, in milk ; ceratin from surface ; mucin in fæces and urine.

Channels of exit of the excreta.

Of water, salts, carbon in gaseous and in solid forms. Of urea and of other nitrogenous compounds, by the fæces, the urine, the skin and the lungs. (Diagram XIII.)

Quantitative relation between income and outgoings of material. The corporeal balance sheet. (*Table* 25.)

Income : by food and water through alimentary canal. Deduct fæces as strictly dregs, omitting the true excreta of the bowels as in quantity insignificant.

Add oxygen by the lungs.

Outgoings by the three great excretory channels : C by lungs, N and minerals by urine, Water by urine, skin and lungs.

Increased income by food : C and H stored as fat and glycogen, N excreted as increased urea. Weight increased.

Diminished outgoing by less work and less active respiration : increased weight as before from fat. Diminished outgoing from disease of excretory organs; poisoning from accumulation of carbonic acid, from "uræmia," or from "cholæmia."

Increased outgoing by active work; diminished weight, call for increased food.

Diminished income : call upon stored fat and glycogen, emaciation : outgoings husbanded by diminished movement, less frequent respirations, slower and weaker circulation, dry skin.

STARVATION. Effect on fatty tissue, on liver, on heart (*Table* 24): symptoms in muscular weakness, and sleep: hybernation: condition of respiration, pulse and temperature. in starvation. State after death of intestines, liver, gall-bladder, &c.

The balance of health (*Table* 25). Power of readjustment after disturbance.

XIII. DIAGRAM ILLUSTRATING THE BALANCE BETWEEN MATERIAL INCOME AND OUTGOINGS OF THE BODY.

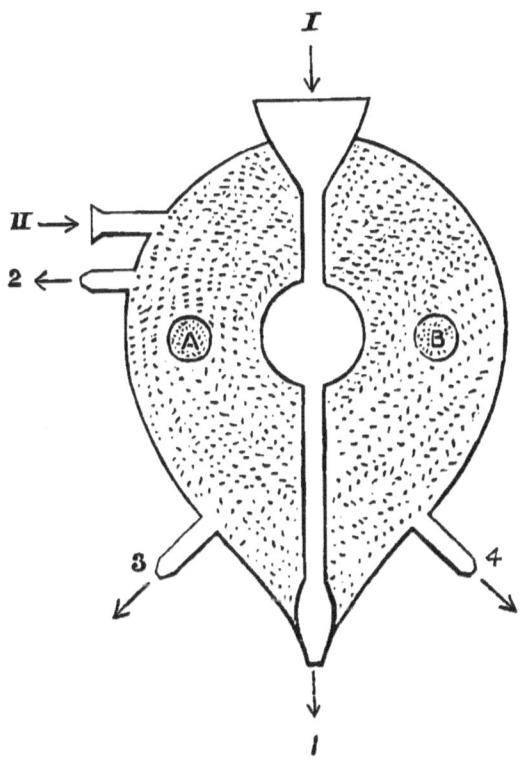

I. Income by mouth of food—proteids, carbohydrates, fats, salts, and water.
II. Income by lungs of air—N and O.
1. Outgoing by rectum of fæces—undigested food, remains of bile, salts, mucus, water, &c.
2. ,, lungs of air—N, O, CO_2, H_2O, &c.
3. ,, kidneys of urine—urea, &c., salts, water.
4. ,, skin of sweat—water, &c.
A. Store of nutriment as fat.
B. ,, ,, ,, glycogen.

To face page 40.

THE WORK OF THE BODY AS A MACHINE.

Source of its energy. Radiant solar heat. Storage of energy in vegetable tissues. Appropriation of latent chemical energy of vegetable proteids, carbohydrates and fats by herbivorous animals: of energy in vegetable and animal compounds by man. This energy rendered kinetic by oxydation, *i.e.* by slow combustion. (*Table* 26.)

Transformation into two forces of energy, *mechanical work* and *heat*. Both dependent (1) on integrity of machine, (2) on supplies of combustible food, (3) on supplies of oxygen; and both regulated by the nervous system.

i. MECHANICAL WORK done by striated and unstriated muscles. Constant work of heart and diaphragm. Production of heat with each contraction. Internal work: mechanical energy transformed into heat by friction.

Relation of outcome of energy as external mechanical work (*e.g.* raising weights) to outcome as external heat, derived partly from internal muscular work as above, and partly from oxydation, which probably accompanies all activity of tissues; pre-eminently muscles, but also glands, nervous centres, and all living protoplasm.

Modes of measuring the income and outgoings of energy. Experimental determination of possible *energy in foodstuffs* by complete combustion into CO_2, H_2O, and NH_3. Deduction of the energy contained in the excreted urea (*Table* 27). Approximate estimation of mechanical *work* done in a day's labour, *e.g.* treadmill, or ascending a mountain. Estimate of work done by the heart. Measurement of *heat* given off from an animal placed in a water chamber—calorimetry.

Units of mechanical energy: the British foot-pound (or

ton) and the Centigrade grammeter (or kilogrammeter). Units of thermal energy: the British pound degree, F°, and the cubic-centimeter degree, C°. Determination of their exact relation, "the mechanical equivalent of heat," by Joule. (*Table* 26.)

ii. HEAT. Bodily temperature approximately constant in health. Result of balance of production and dissipation of heat. Heat produced by oxydation; not in lungs, nor in blood, but in active tissues. Most in liver, next in muscles, least in passive organs, as bones. Heat carried throughout the body by the blood. Heat dissipated on the surface.

1. Loss of heat from the *skin* (*a*) by radiation, (*b*) by conduction, (*c*) by evaporation of sweat rendering heat "latent." 2. Loss of heat from the *lungs* (*a*) by evaporation, (*b*) by expiration of warmed air. 3. Loss of heat which has warmed urine, fæces and other *excreta*.

Or, otherwise put, i. Heat expended by *conduction* and *radiation* from uncovered surface; ii. by *evaporation* from skin and lungs; iii. by *warming* inspired *air* and ingested *food* and *water*. (*Table* 28.)

Adjusting Mechanism. Comparison to a greenhouse.

Clinical thermometry. Mode of measuring mean temperature of the body. History: Sanctorius, De Haen, Hunter, John Davy, Currie, Brodie, Roger, Liebermeister, Wunderlich.

Thermometer in axilla (or groin), mouth, rectum: or held in stream of urine.

Diurnal variations of temperature. Pyrexia; febrile temperature; highest compatible with life; paradoxical temperatures; subnormal temperatures. (*Table* 29.)

Balance of income and outgoings of energy (Diagram XIV.).

XIV. DIAGRAM ILLUSTRATING THE BALANCE OF INCOMING AND OUTGOING ENERGY.

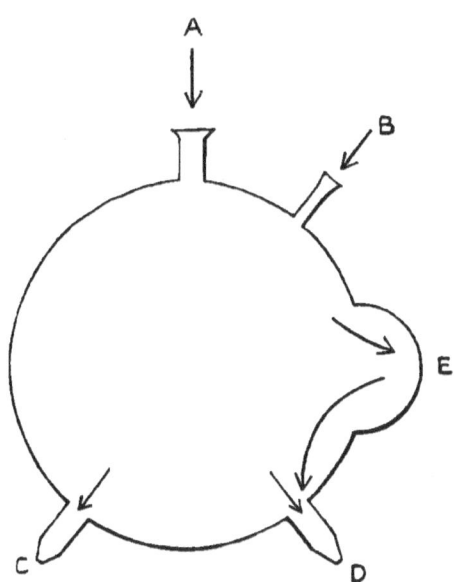

A. Income of energy latent in food.
B. Oxygen admitted by respiration to set free this energy.
C. Outgoing of energy as mechanical movement.
D. ,, ,, heat.
E. Represents the internal movements of the body of which the energy is manifested externally as heat.

XV. DIAGRAMS ILLUSTRATING THE ELEMENTARY COMBINATIONS OF THE NERVOUS SYSTEM.

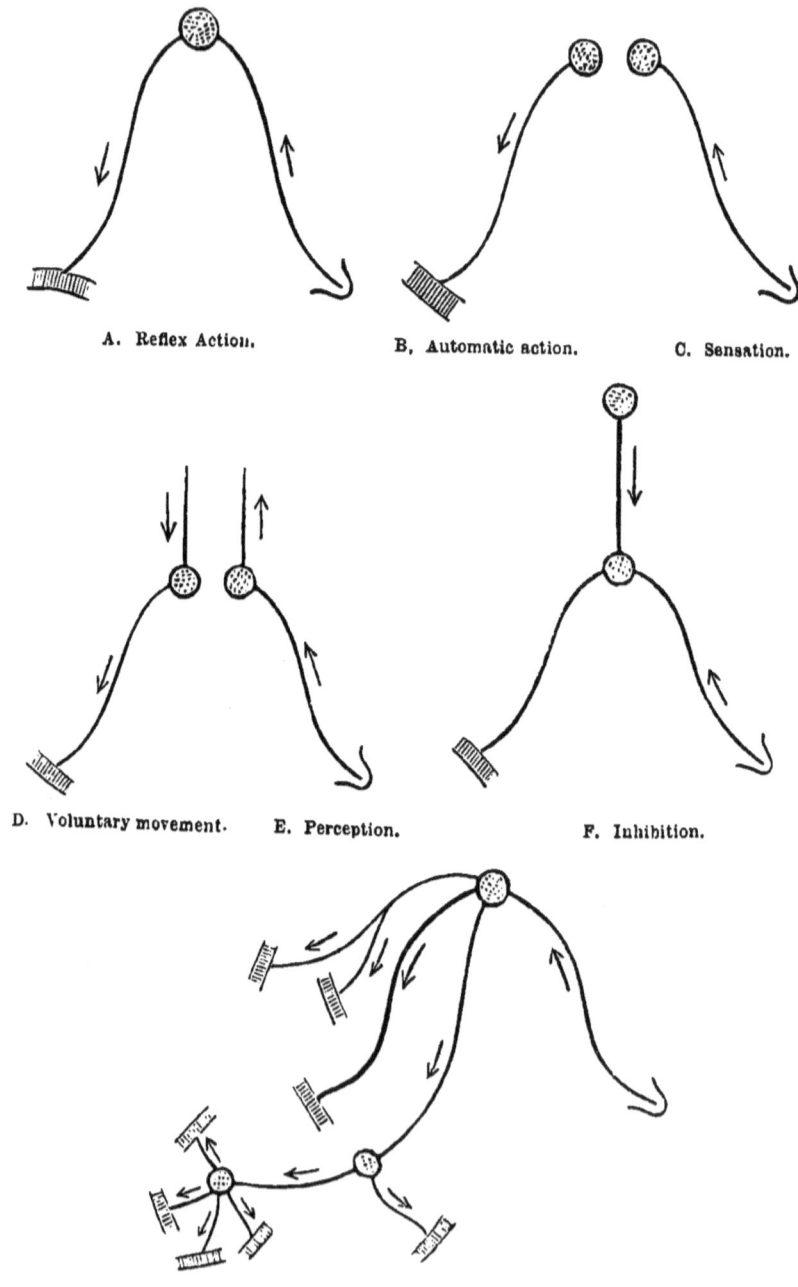

A. Reflex Action.   B. Automatic action.   C. Sensation.

D. Voluntary movement.   E. Perception.   F. Inhibition.

G. Eradiation.

To face page 13.

THE NERVOUS SYSTEM.

Functions of relation with the external world by sensation and movement. Functions associated with mind: consciousness, perception, and will.

Regulating mechanism for secretion, circulation, respiration, and especially for expenditure of energy in muscular movement and heat.

Sensitive surface originally external. Origin of central nervous system in lowest animals by invagination of epiderm, and in the human embryo by invagination of epiblast and subsequent outgrowth from this neural sense-layer.

FUNCTIONS OF THE CONSTITUENT ELEMENTS OF N.S. *Conduction* by Fibres—afferent or centripetal, efferent or centrifugal, and commissural or intercentral. "*Explosion*" or "discharge" of Ganglion-cells following or preceding conduction: "*storage*" by ganglion-cells.

FUNCTIONS OF SIMPLE COMBINATIONS OF NERVOUS ELEMENTS.

End-organ of a sensitive surface, afferent nerve and ganglion-cell. *Sensation* (conscious or no). (Diagram XV., Fig. C.)

Ganglion-cell, efferent nerve and muscle : *automatic movement* (voluntary or no). (Fig. B.)

Afferent nerve, sensory cell, commissure, motor cell, efferent nerve : *Reflex movement* (or secretion). (Fig. A.)

Action of ganglia regulated by *excitant* and *inhibitory* nerves. (Fig. F.) Stimulus, if overstrong, spreads from one to another system : *Eradiation*. (Fig. G.)

Coordination of ganglia of reflex and automatic systems so as to act together in orderly sequence. Theory of co-ordination compared with the mental law of habit. Formation of lines of co-ordination; maintenance, neglect and reinstatement of such lines, compared with learning, practising, forgetting, and recovering a manual art. Inherited habits and manœuvres : the co-ordination of the race. Custom, second nature,* the co-ordination of the individual.

Physiological problem of the Nervous System : the localization of functions in the several ganglia, and the determination of the afferent and efferent (motor, glandular, inhibitory, &c.) tracts between centres and periphery. (*Table* 30.)

Present results of both investigations in order of the anatomical grouping of centres, viz. :—

i. The scattered, so-called "sympathetic," ganglia :— (*a*) cranial, cervical, thoracic, lumbar; (*b*) the visceral ganglia of the heart, of the solar plexus, of the intestines (Auerbach's plexus), of the bladder, and of the genital organs; (*c*) the ganglia on the sensory roots of "spinal" (cranial and vertebral) nerves, including trifacial, glosso-pharyngeal and vagus ; (*d*) the microscopic ganglia of the internal ear and other parts.

ii. The continuous ganglionic sheath which surrounds the "neural tube," including the central canal of the cord, the third and fourth ventricles" and the "aqueduct :" viz. (*a*) grey matter of Cord, or "medulla spinalis," (*b*) do. of Bulb or "medulla spinalis oblongata," (*c*) of Midbrain behind pons, including C. quadrigemina, (*d*) Thalami and C. striata.

iii. Cerebellum.

iv. Cerebral hemispheres.

Methods of determining functions of localized ganglia and paths of conduction. *a. Anatomy* : relations by nerve-fibres to other organs and commissural connection with other ganglia. Histological characters. β. *Comparative anatomy* : degree of development in lower animals in comparison with development of function. γ. *Embryology* : early or later

---

* "By treading the same steps over and over again, they (the animal spirits) presently make a road of it, as plain and smooth as a garden walk, which when they are once used to, the devil himself sometimes shall not be able to drive them off it."—*Sterne*.

appearance: discrimination of nerve tracts afterwards uniform, by absence or presence of myelin (Flechsig). δ. *Experiment.* Ablation or destruction of centres; division of nerves (Magendie, Bell and Joh. Müller, Flourens, Goltz). Stimulation of nerves or centres (E. Weber, Bernard: Fritsch and Hitzig, Ferrier). Degeneration subsequent to ablation or division: (Waller's method; observation of cord and brain after amputations, or excision of eyeball, or olfactory bulb). ε. *Experiments* of disease. Tumours or other destructive affections of centres; secondary ascending and descending degenerations.

i. Functions of the SCATTERED GANGLIA of the "Sympathetic." Their intimate connection with and apparent dependence on the central grey matter by cranial and spinal nerves. Evidence as to the independent functions of the submaxillary and of the lenticular ganglia. Proof of the functions of the several groups of cardiac ganglia. The intestinal ganglia. Absence of ganglia in ureter. Proof of the trophic function of the ganglia of the posterior nerve-roots.

Nerves of the sympathetic or ganglionic "system." Deficient in white fibres. *Afferent from viscera* or mucous membranes, not subserving conscious sensations under ordinary conditions. *Efferent to unstriped muscular fibres* in hollow viscera, or in blood-vessels—vaso-motor nerves. Evidence as to function of cervical sympathetic, of splanchnic, &c.

ii. *Localization of centres* in the GREY MATTER surrounding the neural canal:—

(a) *Cord.* Motor cells in anterior cornua. Trophic centres. Vasomotor centres. Genital centres, &c.

(b) *Bulb:* floor of fourth ventricle. Centres of hearing, taste, deglutition; of cardiac inhibition, blood pressure (vaso-motor and depressor), respiration, &c.

(c) *Midbrain.* Centres of nerves iii., iv. and vi. and of v. Centres of vision in C. quadrigemina.

(d) *Thalami* (?). Connection with tegmentum, C. quadrigemina, and Corona radiata.

Caudate and *lenticular nuclei*, and *claustrum*. Connection with crusta and C. radiata.

Conduction in "spinal system":—

Motor tract: R. corpus striatum, R. crus (crusta), under pons, R. ant. pyramid, decussation, L. deep lateral column, L. ant. cornu, L. ant. nerve root.

Sensory tract: R. post. nerve root, L. lateral column and L. grey matter, L. restiform body (?), L. tegmentum, L. thalamus (?).

R. ant. med. column (Türck) direct to R. crus.

Superficial lateral column direct to cerebellum.

Antero-lateral columns commissural between segments of cord (?).

Posterior columns (Burdach), restiform bodies, cerebellum and thalamus (?).

Post. med. column (Goll), post. pyramids.

iii. CEREBELLUM. Functions unknown.

Pons or transverse commissure. Pr. e cerebello ad testes, or sup. commissure to midbrain. Pr. e cerebello ad med. spin. obl., or inf. commissure to post. columns of cord.

iv. OLFACTORY LOBES. Outgrowth from forebrain with prolongation of ventricle. Nerves from organ of smell. Commissure to C. striatum and cerebrum.

v. CEREBRUM. Outgrowth from sides and front of forebrain, enclosing ventricles continuous with neural canal. Commissural fibres with C. striatum and thalamus, called corona radiata and ext. and int. capsules. C. callosum or transverse commissure. Fornix or longitudinal arched commissure.

Development and comparative anatomy of hemispheres. Fissure of Sylvius. Sulci of Rolando, parieto-occipital, intraparietal, parallel, calcarine, collateral and calloso-marginal. Principal and secondary gyri.

Vascular distribution. Histological differences. "Motor region" of volitional centres. Centres of vision and of other perceptions. Centre of articulation. Discrepancies of observation and interpretation.

XVI. THE PROJECTION SYSTEM.

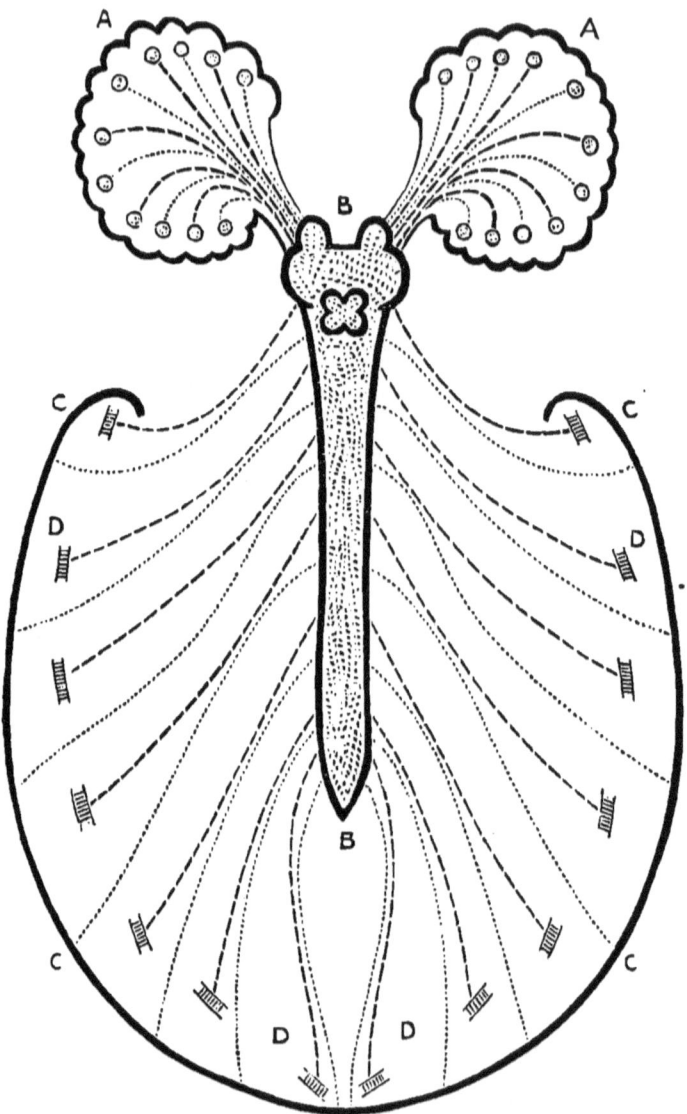

A A. Perceptive sensory, and voluntary motor, centres in hemispheres.
B B. Sensory and motor centres in spinal system.
C C. Sensory peripheral points.
D D. Muscles and other efferent end organs.

NERVOUS SYSTEM. 47

Instances of the practical value of a knowledge of cerebral localization in diagnosis and treatment.

Relation of automatic movement to voluntary movement, to the Will, and the sense of Space: of sensation to Perception: of reflex action to Emotion: of repeated discharge of ganglia to Memory.

Boundary of consciousness not fixed. Some reflex actions perceived. " Unconscious cerebration."

" *The Projection System.*" Necessity for each unit of the sensitive periphery, and for each unit of the muscular periphery, being separately represented in the Hemispheres. Probably also in the grey substance around neural canal (Diagram XVI.).

SPECIAL SENSES.

Efferent end-organs of N.S. motor, electrical (in fishes) or secretory. Afferent end-organs: all modified ectoderm. Origin and gradually increasing complexity. Relation of sensations to perceptions, emotions, and intellect.

Essential parts of a sense-organ: 1. *Epithelial element*, modified so as to be sensitive to only one kind of stimulus or "physical object." 2. Afferent *nerve-fibre*. 3. *Ganglion-cell* in spinal system for sensation. 4. *Commissural fibre* in corona radiata. 5. *Ganglion-cell* in cerebral cortex for perception.

VISION.

Properties of the *physical object*. (See *Note* 31.)

Development of the eye from the midbrain (or forebrain) Primitive optic vesicle with ependyma, ganglion-cells and fibres, and mesoblast, pia mater (choroidea) and dura (sclerotic). Ingrowth of epiderm to form lens, of embryonic corium to form vitreous. Optic cup. Ingrowth of mesoblast: coloboma.

Afferent nerve: chiasma. *Sensory ganglion*, C. quadrigemina and geniculata, with pulvinar of Thalamus. *Percipient centre:* angular gyrus (?).

Orbits, direction of axes. Eyebrows, lids and lashes. Lacrymal apparatus.

Sense-capsule: Sclerotic and Cornea. Anterior chamber, with aqueous humour: a lymph-sinus. Vascular tissue: Choroid and iris: pupil. Refractive media: cornea and aqueous, lens, vitreous. Accommodation: circular "suspensory" ligament or zonule of Zinn, ciliary muscle.

Comparison with a camera obscura.

Formation of images on retina: distinct central and indistinct peripheral vision.

Defects of vision: Muscæ volitantes; Spherical and Chromatic aberration; Astigmatism; Hypermetropia and Myopia; Presbyopia.

Bacillary layer of rods and cones. Proof that they are the true endorgans of vision. Purkinje's figures. The yellow spot and fovea. The ora serrata. *Retinal red* or "vision-purple."

PERCEPTIONS OF VISION—1. *Amount of light.* Comparison of sunlight and artificial light.

2. *Colour.* Nature of physical object. Ultra violet and ultra red rays. Qualities of colour: *a.* "Tone" or hue, primary, secondary, tertiary. Red, green, violet; yellow excluded; claims of blue. Colour-blindness or Daltonism, its degrees and varieties. *b.* "Saturation," intensity or depth. *c.* "Illumination;" amount of white light mingled with colours. "Lustre" or colour seen through a transparent medium which reflects light regularly. Theories of colour perceptions: Young's, adopted by Helmholtz; Hering's.

3. *Form.* Image on retina. No corresponding image in space in brain. System of "signs" between each physical impression and each cerebral excitement. Theory of such "local signs" first propounded by Berkeley.* Combination of sight with touch. Vision with two eyes. Identical points of the R. and L. retinæ.

4. *Solidity and distance.*—Obtained by double vision. Proved by the reflecting stereoscope of Wheatstone, or the

---

* An empirical theory of Vision was taught by Dr. Jurin (a former physician of this Hospital 1684-1750), but the merit of its full exposition is due to Bp. Berkeley, who writes: "That is to say, we perceive Distance not immediately, but by the mediation of a Sign, which hath no likeness to it, or necessary connexion with it, but only suggests it from repeated experience, as words do things." ("Alciphron," vol. i. p. 223.) See also Sect. 88–102 "on erect vision" in his "Essay toward a new Theory of Vision" (1709). The theory of local signs has since been worked out by Lotze.

50 LECTURES ON PHYSIOLOGY.

ordinary refracting one of Brewster. Pseudoscope. Rivalry of the two retinal pictures. "Stereoscopic brilliance."

VISUAL JUDGMENTS. Believing what one sees—its fallacy. Illusions: of form, distance, solidity, illumination, colour, movement. Explanations: by the duration of a visual impression, by comparison or "simultaneous contrast," by retinal fatigue leading to "successive contrast," by experience of diminished size and illumination and colour-tones from distance, by experience of double vision and of perspective effects, by following outlines with the eye, by expectation. Application to the representation of objects by art.

HEARING.

Properties of the *physical object* or stimulus (See *Note* 32).

Development of the ear. *Endorgan*, the modified epidermis lining the auditory capsule, with vibratile bristles (not motor cilia) floating in endolymph. Œdematous connective tissue (perilymph) or modified corium.

Afferent nerve, portio mollis of seventh. *Sensory ganglion* in floor of fourth ventricle. *Percipient ganglion* in posterior part of superior sphenoidal gyrus (?)

Media. Formation of middle ear from first visceral cleft: Eustachian tube, tympanic cavity and external orifice. Subsequent formation of diaphragm (*membrana tympani*) and tympanic ring bone. Chain of tympanic ossicles: *Stapes*, detached from cartilaginous auditory capsule (ossified into petrous or periotic bone), *Malleus* with *pr. gracilis* from proximal end of first visceral arch or mandible. *Incus* with os orbiculare, stapedius and pyramid from summit of second arch. Formation of external ear, auricle, cartilaginous meatus and (after birth) external osseous meatus. Comparison with organ of vision.

Course of sonorous vibrations (*a*) by solids directly through the skull (mastoid pr. or teeth); (*b*) by air through Eustachian tube; (*c*) by membrana tympani, and ossicles vibrating *en masse*. Conduction by external meatus: vibrations of membrane: mechanism of malleo-incudal joints, of the combined lever and its fulcra: probable function of *tensor membranæ tympani* and of *stapedius*. Sonorous vibrations in the perilymph and endolymph.

Structure of labyrinth. Division of primitive auditory sac into two: utriculus and sacculus. Outgrowth of semicircular canals from former, of cochlea from latter. Labyrinth in fishes, and amphibia. Cochlea in birds, monotremes, cetacea, man, rodents. Osseous cochlea, lined with endothelium and filled with perilymph: its two scalæ: use of fenestra rotunda and its membrane to allow vibration in an incompressible liquid. Membranous cochlea (= *scala media* = *canalis cochleæ*), supported on *lamina spiralis ossea*; formed by basilar membrane (= *lam. sp. membranacea*) and Reissner's membrane; lined with modified epithelium from ectoderm; and filled with endolymph. Organ of Corti. Function of Deiter's haircells. Hensen's observations. No special endorgan for musical notes. Semicircular canals probably not auditory (*v. infra* p. 53).

AUDITORY PERCEPTIONS. 1 *Loudness* from amplitude, 2 *Pitch* from length of waves, 3 *Timbre* or "quality" from overtones or harmonics.

Noises and musical sounds: "consonating râles." Duration of impressions: cog-wheels.

AUDITORY JUDGMENTS. 1 *Distance* only from loudness: "ventriloquy." 2 *Direction* only from movement of head or (in animals) of ears.

Memory or recoverability of Auditory compared with that of Visual perceptions. Intellectual importance of the two senses. Emotional power of each.

SMELL.

Physical object: certain substances in state of gas, vapour or suspension in air.

Media absent. *Endorgan* modified epithelium of olfactory capsule (= nasal fossæ in man). *Afferent nerves*, the branches of the first pair. *Sensory ganglion*, the so-called bulbs of the first pair: their structure and development. *Commissure,* the olfactory tract. *Percipient ganglion,* in the unciform gyrus (?).

Relation of odours to oxydation, to chemical composition, to volatility. Smelling by the posterior nares from the mouth, stomach and lungs.

Empirical classification of odours. Their intensity and qualities. Weak memory of odours, and their insignificant intellectual importance. Smell teaches us less of external world than any other senses. Diagnosis of certain diseases by smell: variola, typhus, favus, nutmeg-liver, gangrene of lung, rheumatism. Emotional, and especially sexual, effect of odours in beasts, compared with that of colours and song in birds. The sense almost rudimentary in man.

Taste.

Stimulus: sapid substances in solution. Classification of tastes: sweet, bitter, sour, salt. Many supposed tastes really perceptions of touch, temperature or smell. Relation of taste to chemical composition.

Media absent. *Endorgans* the modified epithelium of the fungiform and circumvallate papillæ and also of fauces and palate. The grooved patches on the rabbit's tongue (papillæ foliatæ). The taste-goblets. Distribution: tip, sides, back of tongue, palate. *Afferent nerve.* The glosso-pharyngeal, its lingual branches: probably not the lingual branch of the fifth, but the chorda tympani of the portio dura (itself perhaps connected at its origin with the glosso-pharyngeal), and the descending palatine branches of the fifth, possibly connected by the great petrosal nerve with the same origin. Sensory and percipient *ganglia* not certainly ascertained.

Perceptions of taste: little recoverable, less intellectual than even those of smell: productive of reflex secretion (salivation) and movement (vomiting): easily fatigued.

Other Senses.

Touch.—*Stimulus;* mechanical pressure. *Medium;* the horny cuticle: raw surfaces without true touch. *Endorgans;*

Corpuscula tactûs and their modifications. *Afferent nerves;* all the fibres which enter by the posterior ganglíated roots of the "spinal" nerves, whether cranial or vertebral—fifth, vagus and first cervical onwards. *Sensory* and *percipient ganglia* less accurately determined for the various sensory surfaces than for any other sense.

Sensations of touch only quantitative. *Distribution.* Weber's method. Tongue, fingers, flexor surfaces, face, limbs, trunk. *Perceptions* recoverable and intellectual, giving the notion of locality. Combination with sight, and with muscular sense.

Ill-defined perceptions, which have their origin in the skin: as *Itching* (especially in healing ulcers), *Tickling* (local distribution), *Formication* or "creeping," *Numbness* (limb "asleep" with blunted touch, from pressure on nerve-trunk; also in Tabes dorsalis), *Tingling* ("pins and needles;" the limb "awaking" after pressure is removed)—all distinguishable from touch, but all more or less pathological or perverted perceptions.

SENSE OF TEMPERATURE. Also with its seat in the skin and mucous membranes: absent in ulcers, lost below pharynx and above rectum. Putting elbow in ice causes cold at the spot and pain in distribution of ulnar nerve. Path of sensory fibres and seat of centre imperfectly known. No quality, only degree appreciated, and extent (hand in basin and body in hot bath). *Distribution,* different from that of touch: tongue, cheeks, lips, palms and soles. *Warmth,* acute or massive perception. *Cold,* in extreme approaches heat as a perception: with exercise, stimulating; without, depressing; reflex effect in rigors.

General, unlocalized, but conscious sensations of *hunger* and *thirst, repletion:* want of *breath,* want of *sleep: fatigue:* want of *muscular movement* after rest: uneasiness from *retained secretions.* Uneasiness (*malaise*) of approaching illness.

Sense of position in space. Evidence of its existence. Probably connected with the semicircular canals. Vertigo. Menière's disease.

Constant influx of unconscious and half-conscious sensations upon the central nervous system both awake and asleep, forming a background for all the more acute and definite perceptions.

MUSCULAR SENSE. Proof of its reality by judging of weights by pressure only and by poising. Its *distribution* and development independent of touch. Larynx (singing), tongue and lips (articulation), fingers (violin-playing, &c.), arms, ocular muscles, legs, trunk. Pleasures of the muscular sense : pains, as fruitless effort (nightmare) and missed blow or step; the former related to the emotion of despair, the latter to that of disgust. Seat doubtful : organs unknown. Probably a central perception of activity of motor ganglion-cells : absent in reflex and other involuntary movements. Intellectual value of the muscular sense : origin of notions of space : Volition.

COMBINATIONS OF SENSES. Sight with touch : sight with muscular sense (of recti) : sight with touch and muscular sense. Smell with taste. Taste with touch, smell and temperature. Touch with muscular sense ("vernier" action).

PAIN. Not a special perception like the above. A mental condition dependent on over-stimulation of any sensory nerve, i.e. excessive stimulation upon a healthy sensorium or ordinary stimulation on a weak and irritable sensorium ("objective" and "subjective" neuralgia). Usual stimulation, pressure ; as by inflammatory exudation, vascular fulness (throbbing), or tumour; or by muscular squeezing (colic and cramp).

Kinds of pain—stabbing, aching, dull, shooting, &c. Degree of pain: estimation by the reflex effect on pupils, on the heart, on blood-pressure, or on the sweat-glands.

Pain antagonistic to perceptions of touch, temperature, and other senses.

Relief of pain by removing pressure or tension, by local or central anodynes, by counter-irritation, i.e. inhibition, by mental and muscular effort, by vocal expiration.

REPRODUCTION AND DEVELOPMENT.

These functions connected with those of nutrition, as vegetative or organic, opposed to animal or relative. Connected with the "animal" function of movement, as also expenditure of matter and of energy. Distinct from both nutritive and animal functions, as concerned not with the life of the individual organism but with the maintenance of the race.

METHODS OF REPRODUCTION. Abiogenesis or *generatio æquivoca*. Its disproof by Redi and subsequent experimenters. *Omne vivum et ovo.**

(1) Non-sexual *fission*, division, segmentation or cleavage.

(2) Non-sexual *gemmation* or budding, either external or internal. Both universal in plants and common in Protozoa, Cœlenterata and Vermes. Absent in Vertebrata and the higher Mollusca and Arthropoda. Non-sexual ovulation or *parthenogenesis* in insects and other invertebrata. Its interpretation. So-called "alternation of generations" or alternation of true generation with non-sexual gemmation or fission.

(3) Sexual reproduction or true *Generation*: fertilization of an ovum or germ-cell (ovule in plants) by a spermatozoon or sperm-cell (pollen-grain in plants.) Probably essentially a checked and modified form of reproduction by fission.

In man, as in other vertebrata, there is no non-sexual reproduction of the entire organism; but reproduction by fission occurs as multiplication of cells in yelk-cleavage, in the embryo, in the growing body, and in disease ("pro-

---

* Nos autem asserimus (ut ea dicendis constabit) omnia omnino animalia, etiam vivipara, atque hominem adeo ipsum, ex ovo progigni.—Harvey: De generatione Animalium. Exercit. I. p. 182 in the College ed. of 1766.

liferation"). Gemmation seen in occasional reproduction of supernumerary fingers after removal ; also in development of fœtal structures in a virgin ovary.

OVULATION. Structure of ovary in man and higher animals (including all vertebrata but osseous fishes) not glandular, but peculiar to itself. Origin and early development of ovary. Its germ-epithelium: its stroma and bloodvessels. Ingrowth of germ-cells in columns. Formation of ova. The ovary and ova at birth. Changes at puberty. Periodical ripening of ova.

The *Ovisac* or Graafian vesicle ("ovum" of de Graaf): its development and structure when fully formed.

Description of the ripe mammalian *Ovum*. Vascular phenomena of menstruation. Application to the ovary of the Fallopian trumpet or oviduct. Rupture of ovisac and escape of ripe ovum. Subsequent changes in ovary: "true" and "false" *Corpus luteum*. Menstruation.

THE SPERM-CELL. Origin, structure, descent, and functional development of testis. Peculiarity of secretion in chemical products being combined with morphological—liquor seminis with spermatozoa. The latter formed by endogenous proliferation in a vacuolated mother-cell (cf. Protomyxia, flagellated infusoria with large nucleus and scanty protoplasm).

IMPREGNATION or fertilization by conjunction of sperm- and germ-cells. Hermaphrodite animals, diœcious and monœcious plants, unisexual flowers. Mutual fertilization even in bisexual organisms. Sexual congress in fishes, amphibia, mammalia.

Place of impregnation normally in upper part of oviduct: extra-uterine pregnancy.

Formation of female pronucleus: extrusion of hyaline polar vesicles or directive corpuscles: radiate appearance of surrounding protoplasm ("aster"). Penetration of zona pellucida by spermatozoa: loss of flagellum and formation of male pronucleus. Conjugation of pronuclei. Description of impregnated ovum.

SEGMENTATION or germ-cleavage. Fission of nucleus:

dumb-bell form: double radiate form ("amphiaster"): cleavage-disk. "Caryolytic figures." Fission of protoplasm. Two equal cells. Repetition of the process. *Morula* or mulberry-mass of segmentation cells. Cleavage cavity. Growth of morula and aggregation of cells towards surface. *Hollow blastosphere* (blastodermic vesicle) with single layer of cells (blastoderm) inclosing segmentation-cavity filled with food-yelk.

Other modes of segmentation according to proportion of living protoplasmic germ and food-yelk or "deutoplasm" in ovum. Ova of osseous fishes, of sharks and skates, of frogs, snakes, and lizards, alligators and tortoises, birds, mammals. Size of ovum dependent on food-yelk. Envelopes albuminous (rabbit, bird, &c.), membranous, calcareous. Complete and incomplete cleavage (*holoblastic* and *mesoblastic* ova): Amphioxys, frog, mammal: osseous fish, reptile and bird (*Table* 33). Structure of hen's ovum. Mode of segmentation: flat disc-like germ, blastodisc or germinal-disc. Its subsequent growth.

Blastoderm or segmented germ. One layer (*epiblast*): size, shape and transparency of constituent cells. Under-cells, large, ovoid, granular: formation of *hypoblast*: two-layered blastoderm. Formation of *mesoblast*: three-layered blastoderm.

FURTHER DEVELOPMENT OF BLASTODERM. Area germinativa. A. pellucida. A. opaca.

Primitive streak and groove; relic of blastopore (?). Medullary or neural groove and canal: laminæ dorsales: incomplete roofing in: hind, mid, and fore neural (cerebral) vesicles: central neural canal and ventricles.

Area vasculosa. Punctum saliens. Primitive tubular heart: primitive or vitelline or omphalo-mesenteric circulation; its partial persistence as vena portæ and affluents.

Head and tail folds: lateral folds. Pinching off of embryo from yelk. Formation of primitive alimentary canal. Fore, mid, and hind gut. Vitelline duct. Yelk sac or umbilical vesicle.

LECTURES ON PHYSIOLOGY.

Formation of cœlom or body cavity. Splitting of mesoblast: limits, cephalad and caudad. Closed pleuro-peritoneal space: a great lymph-sac. Endothelium. Somatopleure and Splanchnopleure.

Notochord. Protovertebræ. Limbs. Development of the several organs from the three layers of the blastoderm (*Table* 35).

Formation of *Amnion* from Epiblast. Internal layer or amnion proper with subamniotic liquor amnii. External layer or "Chorion."

Formation of *allantois* from hindgut. Bladder, urachus and external allantois. Allantoic vessels. Incorporation with "chorion."

Evolution of uterus after impregnation. Muscular fibres: arteries, sinuses. Mucous membrane: decidua: muciparous glands: uterine " milk : " uterine crypts.

Formation of villi over ovum (*Chorion frondosum*). Implantation in uterine crypts. Fœtal and maternal placenta. Allantoic (umbilical or " fœtal-placental ") arteries and vein.

Degree of union of fœtal and maternal elements of placenta. Caducous or non-caducous mucous membrane. Deciduate or non-deciduate placenta.

Form of placenta. Diffuse, *i.e.*, chorion frondosum scarcely differentiated. Zonular and zonary. Cotyledonous. Bell-shaped. Discoid. Placenta and chorion leve.

FŒTAL PHYSIOLOGY.—*Nutrition* : from mucus—uterine milk? —albumen—food-yelk, directly through vitelline duct and indirectly through vitelline veins. From maternal blood. No digestive ferments secreted. Storage of fat and of glycogen. *Circulation*—Fœtal heart: ductus arteriosus and foramen ovale, liver, ductus venosus and umbilical vein. *Respiration*. Diffusion of gases in placenta ; distribution of aerated, unaerated and mixed blood. Expansion of lungs at birth. *Secretion*. Meconium: smegma: urine. *Balance* of nutrition and of energy. Fœtal movements.

Chronology of the chick in the egg and of the human fœtus in utero (*Tables* 34 and 35.)

APPENDIX

OF

NOTES AND TABLES.

NOTES AND TABLES.

1. THE TERM PHYSIOLOGY.

This word occurs in classical Greek in its original meaning of the science, discipline or reasoned discourse, concerning nature —natural philosophy in the widest sense. So φυσιολογία and φυσιολόγος and their derivations were used by Aristotle and Plutarch, and also by Cicero: "*naturæ ratio quam physiologiam Græci vocant*" (de Nat. Deorum, i. 8).

"Physiologus" was the title of one of the most popular books of the middle ages (8th-14th cent.) in the sense of "The natural historian;" but already natural history was chiefly concerned with animals, and the French translation was named "Le bestiaire." The author is unknown. Beside Greek, Latin and Oriental versions, it was twice translated into English. 17 beasts are enumerated, including mermaids, 14 birds, 8 reptiles, and 2 insects, beside a few trees and minerals. See Carus: Geschichte der Zoologie, pp. 108-145.

" Physiology " was used in the general sense of Natural Philosophy by Boyle about 1670, and even a hundred years later Johnson defines it as " The doctrine of the constitution of the works of nature." But I find the word in its modern acceptation of an account of the uses of the parts of the body, in Browne's "Institutions in Physick," London, 1714: and Haller in the middle of the 18th century applies it as we now do.

2. CLASSIFICATION OF THE SCIENCES.

A. *Ideal or Abstract Sciences: subject matter, forms of thought.*

I. MATHEMATICS.
Conceptions of space—Geometry.
Conceptions of number—Arithmetic.
The science of number applied to forms in space—Algebra, &c.

II. LOGIC—the science of the laws of reasoning.

III. METAPHYSICS—the science of real existence.

B. *Real or Material Sciences: subject-matter, sensible objects.*

i. *Descriptive Sciences: "Natural History."*

I. ASTRONOMY, as a science of observation.
II. GEOLOGY and physical geography (*Erdkunde*).
III. MINERALOGY and metallography.
IV. Descriptive BIOLOGY.
Botany.
Zoology.
Anthropology.
Anatomy—Histology—Embryology.

ii. *Exact Sciences: "Natural Philosophy."*

I. PHYSICS: dealing with masses of matter at rest or motion: statics: dynamics.
II. MOLECULAR PHYSICS.
Dynamics of radiant energy—Electricity—Magnetism.
III. CHEMISTRY: dealing with atoms.

iii. *Applied Sciences.*

I. ASTRONOMY : applied mathematics and physics.
II. THEORY OF THE EARTH : applied physics and chemistry.
III. INORGANIC CHEMISTRY.
IV. PHYSIOLOGY: application of physics and chemistry to organic functions. Vegetable—Animal—Human physiology.

Comte's "hierarchy of the sciences" is as follows:

MATHEMATICS.
ASTRONOMY.
PHYSICS.
CHEMISTRY.
BIOLOGY.
SOCIOLOGY.

This classification (founded on the earlier attempt of Descartes) is, as Mr. Herbert Spencer has shown, unsatisfactory in that it compares "Sciences" of different kinds—abstract and concrete.

Spencer's own classification is into :

(1) *Abstract Sciences :* Logic and Mathematics ;

(2) *Abstract Concrete Sciences:* Mechanics ; Molar (including Statics and Dynamics) and Molecular (including Chemistry and the Dynamics of Light, Heat and Magnetism) ;

(3) *Concrete Sciences :* Astronomy, Geology, and Biology.

3. CHARACTERS OF THE ORGANIC KINGDOM.

1. *Chemical*
    Few elements : complex combinations.
    Carbon compounds.
    Colloid condition: abundant water: rounded forms.
2. *Structural*
    Cells and their derivatives: differentiated tissues, neither amorphous nor crystalline.
    Symmetry : spiral, radial, bilateral, serial.
3. *Functional*
    Cycle of changes.
    Origin from a parent organism : growth : assimilation : decay: death.
    Irritability : movement: heat.
    Reproduction.

---

4. DISTINCTIVE CHARACTERS OF ANIMALS AND PLANTS.

1. *Chemical*
    A. predominance of N compounds.
    P.   „   starchy do.   Cellulose tunic to each cell.
    A. Presence of Hæmoglobin.
    P.   „   Chlorophyll.
2. *Structural*
    A. Digestive cavity.   Nervous and muscular tissues.
3. *Functional*
    P. Nutrition from inorganic food.   Fixation of C.
    A.   „   „   organic food only.
    A. Functions of relation predominant.

NOTE.—The group of Fungi form exceptions to many of the above characters: (1) in being without chlorophyll and feeding on organic food; (2) in having a large amount of N and deficient carbohydrates. Carnivorous plants live partly on organic food. A few animals contain chlorophyll—*e.g.*, *Hydra viridis*.

APPENDIX OF NOTES AND TABLES. 65

5. ANATOMICAL CHARACTERS PECULIAR TO MAN.

The distinctions between Man and the lower animals, so far as structure goes, are not of ordinal value, as Cuvier held (*Bimana*), still less of subregnal importance (Owen: *Archencephala*).

Excluding the Lemurs and their allies, as a separate order (*Prosimiæ*), the order *Primates* includes the varieties of the human race—which form a single species, genus and family—along with the families of apes. The group of catarrhine apes which approaches nearest in structure to man consists of the gorilla and chimpanzee (*Troglodytes*), the orang (*Simia* or *Pithecus*), and the gibbons (*Hylobates*).

The characters of the hair, skull, teeth, vertebræ, pelvis and tarsus, of the muscles, the brain and the genital organs, which distinguish man, are given in Huxley's "Anatomy of Vertebrate Animals," pp. 488-492, also by Mivart ("Lessons in Anatomy," p. 494) and Macalister ("Morphology of Vertebrate Animals," p. 334).

The comparative shortness of the forearm, the non-opposable great toe and truly plantigrade foot, the large and completely convoluted brain, the smooth adult skull and large facial angle —are the most striking external human characters.

The permanently erect attitude, and the possession of articulate speech are more important functional peculiarities.

But the deep and broad distinction between man and brutes is intellectual and moral, not corporeal; for, as Bacon remarked long ago: "Man is of kin to the beasts by his body, and if he be not of kin to God by his spirit, he is a base and ignoble creature'

F

6. DEFINITIONS OF DISEASE.

Many and futile have been the attempts to define Health or its opposite, Disease. Both are subjective terms, and therefore not definable by precise predicates, but applied in accordance with individual feeling.

"Disease" is "discomfort." Whatever causes bodily uneasiness or whatever by experience will sooner or later cause it, whatever interferes with our bodily functions, whatever tends to death, is disease. Health is the opposite condition, of comfort, ease, and ability to eat, sleep, move and perform the other functions of life.

Diseases have only this in common, that they all interfere with comfort or shorten life. There is no common cause for the pains of inflammation, of colic and of mechanical injury.

No line can be drawn between health and disease. Pathology is only physiology under various disturbing causes. Decay and death are as much physiological events as birth and life.

All diseases imply two things—an existing cause, *quidquid irritans*, mechanical, thermal, chemical, parasitic, infective, or of unknown nature; and a reacting, living organism, *quidquid irritabile*. Stone in the bladder is not the disease; the disease is the reaction of the body. The severest injuries, the most virulent poisons, produce no disease in a corpse.

There is a tendency after disturbance to return to the previous condition, if the equilibrium has not been too violently upset. This tendency has been called *Vis medicatrix Naturæ*; but there is no such force, and the so-called "efforts of Nature" often aggravate instead of curing the mischief. Our mortal bodies are not made to last for ever.

It is clear that if disease is not a single state nor the result of a single cause, it cannot be removed by any single method, or on any universal principle.

Hence all "Systems" of Medicine, like all "Universal remedies," are of necessity false. Iatro-mechanical and iatro-chemical schools, Brunonian and Antiphlogistic theories, Allopathy and Homœopathy, are all equally unreasonable; not

APPENDIX OF NOTES AND TABLES. 67

wrong solutions of a scientific problem, but ignorant answers to an absurd question.

The rational physician investigates each case of disease to ascertain its seat, its nature, and, if possible, its cause, and treats it accordingly—*Ιατρεύει γὰρ καθ' ἕκαστα.*

7. OBSERVATIONS AND EXPERIMENTS ON ONESELF.

γνῶθι σεαυτόν.

Compare weight, height, and girth of chest.
Ascertain weight of solid food and amount of water daily taken.
Temperature of body on rising, after food, at 8 P.M., and at 6 and 9 A.M.*
Pulse, radial, popliteal, digital. Sphygmographic tracing.
Cardiac impulse, its variation with respiration and with posture.
Respiratory movements, seen in a glass and measured by a tape.
Auscultation (with flexible stethoscope)
   of respiratory pulmonary murmur, of bronchial and tracheal sounds : of cardiac sounds : of bruit musculaire.
Reaction and chemical characters of saliva.
Reaction of sweat.
Quantity, reaction and specific gravity of urine—in hot and cold weather, after sleep, after food, after vegetable diet.
Laryngoscopic examination (on one another). Production of nasal and other consonants.
Difference of height at beginning and end of day.
Expansion of foot in standing and of hand in grasping.
Knee-jerk and superficial and deep reflex movements } on
Relative sensibility to touch and temperature of } one
various parts of skin } another.
Movements of pupil to light, to accommodation. Purkinje's figures. Optical illusions as to form, light, colour.

---

* The most convenient way of rapidly taking the body temperature is to place the bulb of a thermometer in the stream of urine during micturition.

8. CONSERVATION OF ENERGY.

Force is defined as *whatever causes or alters movement;* Energy, as the *power of doing work.*

Forces are numerically estimated by the amount of motion they can produce or destroy in a unit of time—*i.e.,* by the rate at which they can alter motion.

Work is measured by the product of the force acting into the distance moved through.

The several kinds of energy, mechanical, chemical, thermal, electrical, are co-related—*i.e.,* each is capable of conversion into another. Energy is supposed to be, like matter, indestructible. Machines only use existing energy by transforming or applying it—*e.g.,* steam-engine, heat to motion : match, chemical energy to heat and light : battery, chemical to electro-motive energy.

Benj. Thompson (Count Rumford) first showed that the heat produced by friction is proportioned to the mechanical energy employed. Oersted discovered how magnetism may be got out of an electrical current. Faraday how an induced electrical current may be got from a magnet. Dr. Mayer, a medical practitioner of Heilbronn, expounded the theory of conservation of energy. Joule, of Manchester, determined the mechanical equivalent of heat.

There is every reason to believe that vital energy is transformed chemical energy, taken in with food in a latent state and made kinetic in the two correlated forms of energy, heat and motion. And the chemical energy of food is the radiant energy of the sun's rays, rendered latent by the leaves of plants. So that the human body may be regarded as a machine for rendering latent energy kinetic : *i.e.,* for setting free the energy locked up in the complex molecules of starch, oil and albumen, by breaking them down into the simpler and more stable molecules of water, carbonic acid and urea. Energy is thus liberated, and appears as heat and movement.

APPENDIX OF NOTES AND TABLES. 69

9. THE VISCERAL OR BRANCHIAL ARCHES, CLEFTS AND NERVES.

I. *Lacrymal cleft*
Between frontal and nasal arches.
Supplied by first div. of trigeminal nerve.

II. *Nasal cleft*
Between nasal and maxillary arches.
Supplied by bifurcation of oculo-motor or "third" nerve.

III. *Oral Cleft*
Between maxillary (including præ-maxilla, maxilla, palatine, and pterygoid) and mandibular arches.
Supplied by bifurcation of trigeminal nerve or "second and third division of fifth."

IV. *Tympanic (or spiracular) cleft with Eustachian tube*
Between mandibular and hyoid arches.
Supplied by bifurcation of portio dura.

V. *First Branchial or second post-oral cleft*
Between hyoid and thyro-hyoid arches.
Supplied by bifurcation of glosso-pharyngeal.

VI.—VIII. *Second, third and fourth branchial clefts*
Supplied by successive branches of vagus.

10. TABLE OF THE BONES, WITH THEIR HOMOLOGUES.

VERTEBRAL AXIS (*columna spinalis*).

Cervical vertebræ : without ribs reaching the sternum.
Thoracic or dorsal : with ribs attached.
Lumbar : thoracic vertebræ without ribs.
Sacral or pelvic : vertebræ united with ilia, with any others anchylosed with them (as in human sacrum).
Caudal: free post. pelvic vertebræ, called *coccygeal* in man and anthropoid apes.*

SKULL.

Consisting of (1) the *central axis*, formed by the prolongation of the notochord and its sheath; an investing cartilaginous mass, prolonged beyond the end of the notochord in the post. clinoid prs. and incorporating with it the trabeculæ cranii; (2) a series of *neural* (dorsal) *arches* forming the vault; (3) a series of *visceral* (ventral) *arches* forming the jaws, and hyoid and branchial cartilages; (4) external *splint-bones*; (5) three *sense-capsules* wedged in between the segments.

---

* THE PARTS OF A VERTEBRA ARE NAMED AS FOLLOWS :—

Centrum or body: the ossified notochord, or rather its sheath.
Invertebral substance : the unossified notochord.
Neural or *dorsal arch :* pedicles, laminæ and spine.
Hæmal arch : chevron or V-bones (absent in man).
Superior transverse processes, or Diapophyses : post. tubercles of cervical tr. prs. and tr. prs. of dorsal vertebræ.
Inferior do. or Parapophyses ; ant. tubercles of cervical tr. prs. and tr. prs. of lumbar vert.=cervical and lumbar anchylosed ribs.
Anterior zygapophyses—sup. articular prs.
Metapophyses, or mammillary prs.
Posterior zygapophyses—inf. articular prs,
Anapophyses, or post-zygapophyses.

i. POSTERIOR SEGMENT

 Basioccipital............ basilar process.
 Exoccipitals .... condyles.
 Supra-occipital......... squama.

 Auditory capsules

  Periotic or *petrosal* ... petrous part of temporal.
  Tympanic .... ring for membrana tympani.
  Squamosal............... squamous part.
  Malleus .... proximal end of mandibular arch.
  Incus .... proximal end of hyoid arch.
  Stapes or columella ... segment of capsule.

ii. MIDDLE SEGMENT

 Basisphenoid............ posterior part of body.
 Alisphenoids .... greater wings.
 Parietals .... parietal bones.

 Optic Capsules

 Fibrous *Sclerotic*, with osseous plates in birds.

iii. ANTERIOR SEGMENT

 Præsphenoid .... anterior part of body.
 Orbitosphenoids ...... lesser wings.
 Frontals .... frontal bone.

 Olfactory capsules

  Ethmo-turbinals...... lateral masses of ethmoid.

iv. FOURTH SEGMENT (?)

 Mesethmoid .... perpendicular plate and vomer.
 Nasals .... nasals.

 SERIES OF INFERIOR OR VENTRAL ARCHES

1. First or *præ-maxillary*
 ventral arch .... incisor nucleus.
2. *Maxillary* arch with *Jugal* superior maxilla and zygoma.
3. *Palatine* arch .... palate bones.
4. *Pterygoid* arch............... internal pterygoid processes.
5. *Mandibular* arch .... inferior maxilla and malleus
   (*os quadratum*).
6. *Hyoid* arch .... hyoid, lesser process, stylo-hyoid
   ligaments, styloid pr., incus.

THORAX.

Vertebral ribs	bony ribs.
Sternal ribs	costal cartilages.
Præsternum or rostrum ...	manubrium.
Episternum or inter-clavicle	part of clavicle (?) with interclavicular ligament.
Mesosternum	gladiolus.
Xiphisternum	ensiform cartilage.

LIMBS.

UPPER.   LOWER.

1. *Shoulder-girdle*   answers to *Pelvis*.

Scapula	,,	Ilium.
Supra-scapula (epiphysis)	,,	Supra-ilium (epiphysis).
Coracoid bone (anchylosed)	,,	Ischium.
Clavicle	,,	Poupart's ligament. *

2. *Upper arm:* humerus   ,,   *Thigh:* Femur.

3. *Forearm:* ulna   ,,   *Leg:* Fibula.
           radius   ,,   Tibia.

4. *Manus*   ,,   *Pes*.

Radiale or scaphoid	,,	Tibiale } Astragalus.
Intermedium or lunar	,,	Intermedium }
Ulnare or pyramidale or cuneiform	,,	Calcaneum.
Centrale (absent in man)	,,	Navicular or scaphoid.
Carpale i. or Trapezium	,,	Tarsale i. or Entocuneiform.
ii. or Trapezoides	,,	ii. or Mesocuneiform.
iii. or Magnum	,,	iii. or Ectocuneiform.
iv. & v. or Unciform	,,	iv. & v. or Cuboides.
Metacarpals and phalanges	,,	Metatarsals and phalanges.

11. TABLE OF THE ELEMENTS IN THE HUMAN BODY.

C 12 tetrad — in proteids, fats and carbohydrates, as carbonic anhydride and as carbonates.
N 14 triad — in proteids, in crystalline compounds and as a gas.
H 1 monad — in proteids, fats and carbohydrates and as water.
O 16 diad — in proteids, fats and carbohydrates as oxyhæmoglobin, as a free gas and as water.

S 32 diad — in proteids, in a few crystalline compounds and as sulphates.
P 31 pentad — in lecithin and as phosphates.

Cl 35·5 monad — as chlorides.
F 19 monad — as calcic fluoride, probably in form of apatite.

Na 23 monad — as salts, chiefly in liquids.
K 39 monad — as salts, chiefly in solids.
Ca 40 diad — as salts.
Mg 24 diad — as salts.

Fe 56 tetrad — in hæmoglobin and its derivative pigments.

Also a minute but constant amount of Silica in epidermis.

Traces of Manganese with iron, of Lithium with potassium, of Aluminium and of Copper have been detected.

12. TABLE OF PROXIMATE ANIMAL PRINCIPLES.

A. NITROGENOUS

i. Proteids or albuminous compounds.

Albumins
    Serum (or blood) albumin.
    Egg (or ov-) albumin.
    Vegetable albumin.

Globulins
    Serum (or para-) globulin.
    Fibrinogen—Fibrin.
    Crystallin.
    Myosin or muscle-globulin.
    Vitellin or yelk-globulin.

Alkali-albumins—Casein—Legumin, &c.

Acid-albumins—in digestive cavities alone.

Peptones—digested albumins.

ii. Colloid nitrogenous compounds, more or less resembling proteids.

{ *Mucin.*
  Chondrin (?).
  Gelatine.

Elastin, Nuclein, Keratin and other uncertain compounds.

iii. Crystalline proteid body containing iron.
    Hæmoglobin.

iv. Crystalline compounds mostly resembling amides.
    Urea, uric acid, glycin, leucin, tyrosin, &c.

APPENDIX OF NOTES AND TABLES. 75

B. NON-NITROGENOUS

i. Fatty compounds (glycerin ethers).

Palmitin, Stearin, Olein, with traces of *Caproin,* &c.
Lecithin (di-stearyl-glycerophosphate of neurin).
Cholesterin (a monatomic alcohol).

ii. Carbohydrates

Amyloses (ethers)—*Glycogen* or animal starch.
Glycoses (alcohols)—*Dextrose* and *lævulose, Maltose.*
Sucroses (alcohols)—*Lactose.*

13. CONSPECTUS OF THE MOST IMPORTANT CHARACTERS OF THE PRINCIPAL CARBOHYDRATES.

Name.	C	H	O	Water.	Alcohol.	Diff.	Polarised ray.	Iodine.	Copper.	Changed into
Gum (Arabic Acid K & Ca)	6	10	5	sol.	insol.	colloid	—	...	...	—
Cellulose (Lignin).	6	10	5	insol.	insol.	...	...	—	...	—
Starch (Granulose)	6	10	5	"sol."	...	colloid	+	blue (at 80°)	...	glycose.
Animal Starch (Glycogen)	(6	10	5)$_3$	"sol."	insol.	colloid	+	cherry (at 60°)	...	maltose & glycose.
Dextrin ("British gum")	(6	10	5)$_2$	sol.	insol.		+	claret (at 65°)	...	do.
Dextrose (Glycose)	6	12	6	sol.	sol.	cryst.	+	...	reduces	alcohol.
Lævulose (Fructose)	6	12	6	sol.	sol.	cr.	—	...	reduces	do.
Galactose (artificial product)	6	12	6	sol.	sol.	cr.	—	...	reduces	do.
Inosit	6	12	6	sol.	...	cr.	...	...	...	...
Maltose	12	22	11	sol.	sol.	cr.	+	...	reduces	do.
Lactose (milk sugar)	12	12	11	sol.		cr.	+	...	reduces	lactic acid.
Sucrose (cane sugar)	12	22	11	sol.	...	cr.	+			

APPENDIX OF NOTES AND TABLES. 77

14. PFLÜGER'S TABLE

Of the effects of making and breaking a constant Galvanic Circuit, ascending or descending (*i.e.*, centripetal or centrifugal) through a muscle-nerve preparation.

Electro-motive force of battery or number of cells alternately coupled.	Descending Current		Ascending Current	
	Make (closing contr.)	*Break* (opening do.)	*Make* (closing contr.)	*Break* (opening do.)
Very weak.........	Contraction	... None	Contraction	...... None
Weak	Contr.	None	Contr.	None
Stronger......	Contr.	Contr.	Contr.	None
Moderate..........	Contr.	Contr.	Contr.	Contr.
Strong	Contr.	Contr.	None	Contr.
Very strong	Contr.	None or tetanus	None (recoil block)	Contr.

Deductions. A descending current is more efficient than an ascending one. The stimulus of making is more efficient than that of breaking the circuit. Efficiency increases with electromotive force up to a certain point; then blocks interfere. Conductivity of nerve is increased by catelectrotonus and diminished by anelectrotonus.

General Law. Electrical stimulus consists in the passage of nerve or muscle from a lower to a higher state of irritability, *i.e.*, either (1) rise of catelectrotonus or (2) fall of anelectrotonus. Of the two, the former is the more efficient stimulus.

Notation.—The results set forth in the above table are conveniently stated thus : CCC (or KCC) means cathodal (kathodal) closing contraction—*i.e.* on making a descending current, a contraction follows; ACC = anodal closing contraction—*i.e.* on making an ascending current, a contraction follows; COc = on breaking a descending current, a weak contraction; AOO = on breaking an ascending current, no contraction; COT = on breaking a descending current, tetanus.

15. LAWS OF DIFFUSION OF LIQUIDS THROUGH MEMBRANES.

Crystalline solutions diffuse better than colloid.
Acid solutions better than neutral.
Aqueous solutions better than oily liquids.
With two diffusible solutions the greater current is from that of less to that of greater specific gravity.
The membrane must be "wetted" by the liquid. Hence soaps facilitate the passage of oils.
Difference of pressure on the two sides of the membrane modifies the above rules.

16. COMPARISON OF LYMPH, CHYLE AND BLOOD.

	Lymph (interstitial in connective tissue).	Lymph (between lymph glands and veins).	Chyle (in Receptacle).	Blood.
Reaction......	neutral or alkaline	alkaline	alkaline	alkaline
Sp. gr..........	little above 1000	1015–1020	1015	1055
Water..........	nearly the whole	950	900	800 (pro mille)
Salts...........	·5	7	7	8
Albumin / Globulin	trace	35	40	70
Fibrin	absent	·5	2	2·5
Fatty matter	trace	5	35	1
Leucocytes ...	few or absent	abundant	more so...	less abundant
Red disks......	absent	absent	absent	about 4 millions to each square millimetre

APPENDIX OF NOTES AND TABLES. 79

17. PHYSICAL LAWS AFFECTING THE CIRCULATION.

1. Gravity—*Weight* of the blood. *Inertia* of the blood; of the vessels. Weight of air—*atmospheric pressure*.

2. Blood (like water) almost absolutely *incompressible* and inelastic.

3. Blood (like water) *transmits pressure equally* in every direction,—*i.e.*, the molecules of a liquid move freely among each other.

4. Blood, under pressure, *moves in the direction of the least resistance*.

5. *Friction* of liquid moving in closed tubes: external between wall and liquid, internal between layers of liquid (the latter may be neglected). Effect in causing a slow current externally and the most rapid in axis of tube. (Current of a river slowest near banks, swiftest in mid-stream.)

6. *Quantity* of a given liquid discharged in a given time from tubes depends (1) on the average velocity of the whole stream, (2) on the calibre of the tube—*i.e.*, the square of the radius multiplied by π ($\frac{22}{7}$ or $3\cdot1415927$), (3) on the length of the tube.

7. The *Velocity* varies (neglecting friction) as the moving energy (*vis viva*). It may be measured by the difference of pressure at the two ends of the tube, if the latter is less than $0\cdot5$ mm. in diameter. Where the moving force, like the contraction of the heart, is intermittent, the velocity varies with its energy and frequency—*i.e.* as the mean pressure at the proximal end of the tube varies.

8. *Friction* for the same liquid (blood) and same surface (healthy endothelium) depends on the length of tube traversed, and (for a capillary tube) on the square of its cross-section.

9. *Elasticity* of the tubes probably makes little difference in the mean velocity, or in the friction, and none in the total amount of liquid discharged in a given time. Its effect is only to equalize the mean pressure and so to convert an intermittent into a more or less constant flow.

18. TABLE OF SUCCESSIVE EVENTS IN A COMPLETE CARDIAC CYCLE.

AURICLES	contracting, B. P. highest	relaxed, B. P. low	relaxed, slowly filling	relaxed	relaxed	relaxed full	relaxed nearly full
VENTRICLES	distended	contracting, B. P. rising	contracted and empty	relaxing, B. P. lowest	relaxed filling		contracting
AORTA AND PULM. ART.	contracted, B. P. lowest	distending, B. P. rising	distended	contracting	contracting		contracting
AUR.-VENT. VALVES	open	shutting	shut	opening	open	open	shut
SIGMOID VALVES	shut	opening	open	shutting	shut	shut	shut
Periods	"Pause" (auricular systole)	"systole"	"systole"	"interval"	"diastole"	"pause"	
Sounds		first sound, impulse			second sound		
Murmurs	presystolic or auriculo-systolic	systolic	systolic	post-systolic	diastolic		post-diastolic

APPENDIX OF NOTES AND TABLES. 81

19. STATISTICS OF THE CIRCULATION.

The Amount of blood in the body is about one 12th or 13th of the entire weight, *i.e.*, for an average man, about 12 or 13 lbs.

Of this about 10 or 12 lbs. are said to escape after decapitation; or 7 or 8 by opening the heart and veins after death. The rest remains in the tissues.

Of the whole quantity, more than a fourth is in the *heart and great vessels*, nearly as much in the *portal system*, including the liver and mesenteric vessels, and most of the rest in the *muscles, glands* and *brain*.

The heart contains in each of its cavities approximately the same amount; which has been calculated at 4, 5 or 6 oz. Ludwig gives 150 c.c., Vierordt 180, Sanderson 195, *i.e.*, 5½–6 oz.

Blood-pressure in *left ventricle* of the horse—during systole—estimated at 200 mm. (8 in.) of mercury; in its *aorta* not much less : 15–20 cm. or 7·5 inches. In its *right ventricle* only 25 mm. (1 in.), and in its *R. auricle* 2-3 mm. In L. ventr. of dog 140 mm. (Marey).

Blood pressure in dog's carotid artery .... 4–7 in.
,, ,, rabbit's ,, ... 2–4 ,,
,, ,, sheep's brachial vein .... ⅛ ,,
,, ,, ,, crural ,, ... ⅓ ,,
Estimated pressure in human carotid .... 6–8 ,,

Mean *velocity* in carotid of horse .... 12 in. per sec.
,, ,, metatarsal of horse .... 2 ,, ,,
,, ,, carotid of dog.................. 10 ,, ,,
,, ,, ,, rabbit .... 5 ,, ,,

According to Chauveau's observations, the rate varies extremely, from 8 to 20 in. per sec. in the horse, and from 8 to 15 in the dog.

Velocity of pulse-wave, 9 metres per sec.

Time for complete circulation—from jugular vein to carotid—in horse reckoned at 30 sec. (Hering : 28 Poiseuille), and in man about the same : in dog 15 sec., in rabbit 7 or 8 sec., in cat the same, fowl 5, squirrel 4 (Vierordt).

APPENDIX OF NOTES AND TABLES.

Pulse per minute: in the fœtus 150
,, infant 130-150
,, child 80-100
,, adult............... 70

but varying from 65 to 80 or more within physiological limits.

In tall persons it is usually rather slow: in old age somewhat quickened.

20. PHYSICAL LAWS AFFECTING RESPIRATION.

Pressure of air (at sea-level), 15 lbs. to square inch.
This pressure *acts equally* in all directions.
Air, like liquids, follows direction of least resistance.
Air *compressible* and *elastic*.
The *volume* varies inversely as *pressure* (Boyle's law) at constant temperatures.
Diffusion of gases—freely.
Transfusion—through animal membranes.
Solubility of gases—varies with barometric pressure.
,, inversely with temperature.

Specific solubility of
  O in serum, at 760 mm. mercury and 0° C. . ·04
  CO_2 . . . . 1·79
  N . . . . ·021
  Atmospheric air . . . . . . ·025

21. STATISTICS OF RESPIRATION.

Total capacity of both lungs, about 400 c.c. of air. Of this about 100 c.c. is only inspired by effort ("complemental" air); about 25 or 30 are changed in tranquil phrenic respiration ("tidal" air); about 100 are only expired by muscular effort ("reserve" air). Of the remaining 150 ("residual" air), some escapes on opening the thorax after death and so equalizing pressure outside and inside the lung; while the larger part can only be expelled by long-continued pressure overcoming the elasticity of the pulmonary tissue.

Quantity of oxygen inspired per diem, with moderate exercise, about 10,000 grains, or nearly 1½ lbs. (745 grammes or nearly 520 litres).

APPENDIX OF NOTES AND TABLES. 83

Quantity of carbonic acid gas expired per diem varies greatly with muscular work. For a day of moderate exercise it has been estimated at 12,000 grains, or from $1\frac{3}{4}$ to 2 lbs. (800–867 grammes): on a day of rest in Pentonville Prison, 911 grammes; on one of enforced labour, 1284.

Quantity of water expired per diem estimated at 11 fl. oz.

Frequency of respirations (while at rest, as in sleep): at birth, 40 per minute; during childhood, 25 per minute; during adult life, 16 or 17 per minute.

Inspired Air.		Expired.	Venous Blood.		Arterial Blood.
N (by vol.) 79	...	79	O (at 30 in.) 9–10	...	20
O 21	...	16	CO_2 46–49	...	39
CO_2 trace	...	4–5	N 2	...	2

22. TABLE OF VOWELS.

Pure vowels:

(1.) I long: as in rav*i*ne, usually in English written *e* as in *E*ve, or *ee* as in eel, or *ea* as in deal.
Short: as in *i*f, also crypt.

(2.) A long: as in f*a*ther, p*a*ss; rare in English and written as *ah*, or *alms*, or star.
Short: scarcely occurs in English.

(3.) U long: as in bl*u*e: usually written *oo* in English as in too soon, also in *two*, *to*, *rule*, *blew*.
Short: as in s*u*gar, f*u*ll, also written *oo* as in look and wolf.

Intermediate vowels:

i. between I and A.

(1.) E long: as in con*vey*, usually in English written *a* as *a*le, mate.
Short: as in then, bell.

(2.) Æ long: as in there, pear; perhaps only ĕ modified by the following r.
Short (German ä) as in m*a*t, *A*lfred (old English Ælfred).

84 APPENDIX OF NOTES AND TABLES.

ii. Between A and U.

(3.) ŒE long: in German ö, in French eu; as in t*u*rn, w*o*rm, h*e*rb, f*i*rst.
Short: as in t*u*n, *u*p.

(4.) A-broad, long: as in *a*we, *ou*ght, p*a*ll, sp*o*rt.
Short: written *o* in English as in p*o*ll, sp*o*t.

iii. Between U and I.

(5.) Ü long and short in German and *u* in French: only provincial in English.

Diphthongs (all long):

(1.) AI usually written *i*, as in b*i*nd, d*ie* : also b*uy*, b*y*, *eye*.
(2.) AU usually written *ou*, as in b*ough*, n*ou*n, also h*ow*, n*ow*.
(3.) OU usually written *o*, as in *o*mega, w*oe*, s*o*le; also *owe*, s*ou*l, l*ow*, b*oa*t.
(4.) OI as in b*oi*l; also b*oy*.

Semi-vowels:

(1.) I short, preceding and coalescing with any other vowel or diphthong: written *y* as in ye, yard, you, yea, yearn, yawn, yacht.
(2.) U short, precedent: written *w* as in wet, worm.

23. TABLE OF CONSONANTS.

	LABIALS (lips and incisors).		DENTALS AND SIBILANTS (tongue and incisors or hard palate).				GUTTURALS (root of tongue and soft palate).	
	mute	vocal	mute	vocal	mute	vocal	mute	vocal
ABRUPT	P	B	T	D	S	Z	K	G
CONTINUOUS:								
resonator open...		M		N				NG
trilled (liquids)...				L		R		
aspirated	F	V	TH (thin)	TH (the)	SH	ZH	CH (loch)	GH (lough)
semivowels		W		...		...	H	Y

Examples. Mutes and vocals are interchanged by Welshmen and by Germans in speaking English.

When the nares are obstructed, M becomes B; N, D; and NG, G.

APPENDIX OF NOTES AND TABLES. 85

That L is related to D is shown by 'Οδυσσεύς becoming *Ulysses*, and δάκρυον *lacryma*.

That R is related to S is shown by dialectic forms like θάρρος for θάρσος and variations such as *arbor* and *arbos*.

The relation of sibilants and dentals is shown by children's talk and by dialectic forms like θαλάττα for θαλάσσα.

The relation of the labials and gutturals and dentals among themselves is shown by forms like *Pater*, *Father*, *Vater*; *Tochter*, *Daughter*, θυγάτηρ; *Tooth*, *Dens*, *Zahn*; *Three*, *Tres*, *Drei*.

W is a weakened V, as heard in vulgar English. H is a weakened CH: thus *Ham* is in Greek χάμ, *hirundo* χελιδών, *hiems* χειμών.

Y is a weakened GH, as in Berlin pronunciation. The old English y as a prefix of a past participle is the German *ge*. So *yawn* is gähnen, *yesterday* Gestern, *yellow* gelb.

THE ENGLISH ALPHABET is both defective and redundant. We have lost the old English signs for the vocal and mute aspirated dentals; þ (th as in *thick*) and ð (th as in *then* absurdly printed and still more absurdly pronounced y in the word *the*. We have no single symbols for the two aspirated sibilants Sh (=German sch) and Zh (=French j) as in *azure*. The aspirated gutturals are not English sounds. CH is the Greek χ and the German *ch*, and the north English dialect retains the sound: e.g., *loch*. GH is the German g-final and appears in the Irish form of the word lake or loch, *lough*.

Redundant letters are C =K or S, J=D Zh, Q=K, X=K S.

The vowels and diphthongs are extremely irregular; A has been generally softened into E, and E into I, while I long has acquired the sound of the diphthong AI. One reason for these anomalies is that, while Southern *pronunciation* has predominated in polite English, many of the *written* forms are Northern.

The *alphabet* (English, Roman, Greek, Phœnician, and Hebrew) is not a haphazard arrangement of signs, but a series of quaternions, containing each a vowel, labial, guttural and dental, thus:—

Vowels	A	E	I	O	U
Labials	B	F(digamma)	M	P	V (phi)
Gutturals	C(gamma)	G	K	Q(koppa)	X (chi)
Dentals	D	(theta)	L N	R S T	Z

24. EFFECTS OF STARVATION.

Results of observations by Chossat and by Voit.

The heart loses least weight, only . . 2–2·5 per cent.
The brain also after death has lost only . 2–3 per cent.
The bones 15
The blood the same as the whole body . . 17–25
Lungs, 17; skin, 20; kidneys, 25–30
Muscles (diaphragm least) . . . . 30–40 per cent.
Liver about half its weight 50–55
Spleen 65–70
Adipose tissue turned into connective tissue
    by losing all its fat, or . . . . 95–97 per cent.

25. BALANCE OF HEALTH.

Income.

Food, 1½–2 lbs.
Water, Oiv, or 5 lbs.
Oxygen gas, 1½ lbs, or about 10,000 grains.
Deduct the undigested matter passed as fæces, about ℥vj.

Outgoings.

By the lungs:
  C (as CO_2) . . . . . 250 grammes, or 7½ oz.
  Water as vapour . . . 330 c.c., or 9 ,,

By the skin:
  Water as sweat and vapour . 660 c.c., or 20 ,,
  Besides trace of salts and N.

By the kidneys:
  Water . . . . . 1700 c.c., or 50 ,,
  Salts . . . . . . 20 gr., or 5 dr.
  Urea . . . . . . 30–33 gr., or 8 ,,

APPENDIX OF NOTES AND TABLES. 87

26. TABLE OF AVAILABLE ENERGY IN ONE GRAMME OF VARIOUS ARTICLES OF DIET.

One gramme (15·4321 grains) of potatoes yields about 1000 (997–1013) gramme degrees C. or Centigrade heat units or "caloris," *i.e.*, it would raise about 1000 c.c. or 1 litre of water from freezing point to 1° C. Or, multiplying by Joule's "mechanical equivalent" of heat 424 we have 424,000, *i.e*, the same energy would lift that number of grammes (or 424 kilograms) one metre.

One gramme			
Dried potatoes yields	3700–3752 thermal units		[meters.
Flour	3850–3950	,,	
Dried white of egg	4998	,,	or about 2000 kilogram-
Dried beef muscle	5313	,,	,, 2250 ,,
Gelatin	4520	,,	,, 1614 ,,
Urea	2205	,,	,, 934 ,,
Starch	3813	,,	,, 1600 ,,
Sugar (dextrose)	3277	,,	,, 1388 ,,
Alcohol	7076	,,	,, 2975 ,,
Palmitin	8888	,,	,, 3768·5 ,,

27. BALANCE OF ENERGY.

Income. Supposing a man to eat 100 grammes of proteids in the shape of lean meat, the same weight of fatty matter as bacon or butter, and 250 grammes of starch as potatoes and arrowroot cooked in various ways, beside the non-oxydisable water and salts, he will be taking in as available energy, on Frankland's reckoning (which differs slightly from the figures given in Table 26), the following.

By meat, 5103 × 100 heat units. But the animal body cannot oxydise proteid food down to CO_2 H_2O and NH_3. The nitrogen is excreted as urea, in bulk about a third of the proteids eaten. Urea has an (unused) energy of about 2206 thermal units. So deduct $\frac{1}{3}$ of this, to allow for the unexhausted energy of the proteids, represented by the urea they are reduced to.

Then the 100 grammes of meat will yield—$(5103-\frac{2206}{3}) \times 100$

or 436,800 heat units

100 grammes of fat will yield 9069 × 100 or 906,900 heat units

And 250 grammes of amyloids 3912 × 250 or 978,000 heat units

2,321,700 thermal units

So that the amount of daily energy taken in, thus estimated, comes to, say 2322 kilogram degrees (= 984,528 kilogrammeters in terms of work). Similar calculations by Fick yielded 2600-2700 kilogram degrees, by Ranke 2200, by Barral 2706, and by Helmholtz 2700.

Outgoings. These cannot be estimated so exactly even in theory. A "day's work" has been reckoned at 450 foot tons, or 150,000 kilogrammeters. But this is only external work. The internal work of the heart, diaphragm, &c., only appears as heat, and we cannot separate this heat of friction from that directly produced by oxydation. The total heat evolved in 24 hours with a fair day's work has been estimated at more than two million heat units—2,061,320 or 2,732,472. See next Table.

28. OUTGOINGS OF HEAT.

1. By warming the air taken in—otherwise put as "by loss of the warm air expired."
2. By warming the food and drink taken in—otherwise put as "by loss of heat in the urine and fæces discharged.
3. By heat becoming latent in evaporation in the lungs and skin.
4. By radiation and conduction from the exposed parts of the body.

The proportionate amounts have been estimated as follows by Barral, Dulong and Helmholtz in (centigrade) thermal units:

	BARRAL.	DULONG.	HELMHOLTZ.
	Per cent.	Per cent.	Per cent.
By warming food ...	52,500 or 2·3	47,500 or 1·8	70,000 or 2·5
By warming air inspired	100,800 or 3·7	84,500 or 3·5	70,000 or 2·5
By Evaporation from lungs	} 700,000 or 25·3	192,000 or 7·2	398,000 or 14·8
By Evaporation from skin		384,000 or 14·5	} 2,000,000 or 80.
By Conduction and Radiation............	1,820,000 or 67·5	1,791,000 or 72	
	2,673,300	2,499,000	2,538,000

APPENDIX OF NOTES AND TABLES. 89

29. TEMPERATURES.

Fahr.		Cent.
230°	Hot dry air has been borne without clothing	110
225	Chamber used by Drs. Blagdon and Fordyce	107·2
212	Water boils at 30 in. (760 mm.) pressure	100
194	Sodium melts	90
	(Lead at 334°, Iron at 1,000° or upwards)	
183	The highest point of coagulation of serum-albumin	84
170	Coagulation of serum-globulin	77
160	Coagulation of ordinary serum-albumin	73 to 70
158–150	Hot air bath	70–65·5
137	Potassium melts	58
131	Stearin melts	55
122–115	Warm-blooded animals die	50–46
115	Observed in scarlatina by Woodman	46·1
112·5	Observed in tetanus by Wunderlich	44·75
111	Normal temperature of the swallow	44
110·3	Highest temperature certainly recovered from	43·5
110–100	Hot bath	43–38
105	Normal temperature of squirrel	40·5
104	High febrile temperature in man; normal in sheep	40
103·5	Blood of hepatic vein (Bernard)	39·7
103	Normal temperature of rabbit	39·5
101·5	Blood of right auricle	38·6
100·5-99·5	Normal temperature of dog	38–37·5
99	Normal temperature in human rectum	37·2
97·5–98·6	„ „ „ mouth	
98·6	„ „ „ axilla	37
95–98	Subnormal temperatures	35–36·7
95–86	Tepid bath	35–30
90°	Ether boils	32·2
60–59	Warm air: cold water: "temperate"	15
60–50	Cold bath	15–10
32	Cold air. Ice melts. Water freezes	0

NOTE.—To turn Fahr.° to C.° subtract 32, multiply by 5, and divide by 9.

To turn C.° into Fahr.° multiply by 9, divide by 5, and add 32.

30. TABLE OF CENTRES AND COMMISSURES.

I. Continuous axial tract of grey matter surrounding the neural canal: viz., grey matter of cord, of bulb, of mesencephalon around aqueduct, and of third ventricle.

Transverse commissures: *white* between anterior cornua of cord.

Longitudinal: *antero-lateral* white columns.

II. Thalami

Transverse commissure: *posterior* of third ventricle.

III. Corpora striata

Transverse commissure: *anterior* of third ventricle in part.

Radiating commissure with cortex of hemisphere: *corona radiata*.

IV. Olfactory Bulbs

Longitudinal commissure to I. and III. (*nervus olfactorius*.)

V. Cortex of Hemispheres

Transverse commissure: *Corpus Callosum*.
Longitudinal arched commissure: *Fornix*.

VI. Cerebellum

Transverse commissure: *Pons Varolii*.
Longitudinal to grey matter of cord: *C. restiformia*.
Longitudinal to grey matter of mesencephalon: *Pr. e cerebello ad testes*.

APPENDIX OF NOTES AND TABLES. 91

31. PHYSICAL PROPERTIES OF LIGHT.

QUANTITY: or extent of illuminated surface in the field of vision, intensity of illumination.

INTENSITY: depends on amplitude of vibrations of ether.

COLOUR: depends on number per second of vibrations of ether. Perceptions of colour depend upon (1) *Tone*, tint, or hue—*i.e.* the actual length of the vibrations; (2) *Saturation* or depth or purity of hue; (3) *Illumination* or brightness, or intensity.

Rays of light move in straight lines, and are reflected or absorbed or transmitted by every object on which they fall.

Partial and total reflexion : regular and irregular reflexion.

Angle of reflexion equal to angle of incidence.

Angle of refraction, different for different transparent media. Index of refraction μ, is the ratio of sine of angle of incidence to sine of angle of refraction.

Value of μ for air to water 133 : 100; to vitreous humour 136 : 100; to aqueous humour 133·8 : 100; for water to lens 145 : 100.

32. PHYSICAL PROPERTIES OF SOUND.

LOUDNESS depends on amplitude of vibrations.

PITCH depends on frequency of vibrations (or number per second).

TIMBRE ("quality") depends on the overtones or harmonics which accompany the ground-tone or fundamental note.

Range of audible sounds from 32 to 73,000 per second.

Conduction of sound best by uniform elastic solids, next by uniform liquids, next by air. Most interrupted by heterogenous combination of solids and liquids, or by layers of solids with air or water between.

33. SEGMENTATION OF OVUM.

i. HOLOBLASTIC: complete, with no separate vitellus or yelksac.

(1.) *Regularly symmetrical throughout ovum:*
Most sponges and polyps.
Ascaris and some other worms.
Most Echinodermi.
Some lower Crustacea.
Podura among Insects.
Chiton among Mollusks.
Amphioxys among Vertebrates.

(2.) *More or less unsymmetrical:*
Rabbit and probably other placental Mammals (very nearly regular).
Frog and other Amphibia and Ganoid fishes.
Most Mollusca, &c.

ii. MEROBLASTIC: incomplete: with separate vitellus and yelk-sac:
Birds and reptiles.*
Sharks and rays.
Osseous fishes.
Cephalopoda } yelk differentiated from germ
Most arthropoda } only after impregnation.

iii. CENTROLECITHAL: with vitellus in centre of blastoderm separate but not inclosed in an external yelksac.

(1.) *With regular complete segmentation:*
Certain crustacea, as Pagurus.

(2.) *with unequal segmentation:*
Certain crustacea, as Gammarus.

(3.) *With surface segmentation and very large yelk:*
Many insects, as Aphis.

* Mr. Caldwell reports, Sept. 1884, that the Monotremata alone among mammals lay a meroblastic ovum.

APPENDIX OF NOTES AND TABLES. 93

34. CHRONOLOGY OF THE EMBRYO CHICK.

The First day of Incubation.

1—12 hours. Hypoblast formed completely.
Mesoblast.
Primitive streak and groove.

12—24 hours. Head-fold.
Medullary or neural groove.
Notochord and protovertebræ.
Mesoblast splits to form the cœlom.
Amnion begins to form.
Area vasculosa.

Second day.

1—12 hours. Medullary or neural canal.
Cerebral vesicle, I. Head-fold.
Tubular heart.
Wolfian duct begins to appear.

12—24 hours. Cerebral vesicles, II. and III. Eye and ear sacs.
First circulation. Tail-fold.
Amnion completed.

Third day.

Embryo turns on to left side.
Cranial flexure.
Visceral clefts and arches.
Lens and eye-cup. Fore and hind gut. Lungs and liver.

Fourth day.

The invaginated mouth or stomodœum opens into the fore-gut.
The allantois is formed.
The septum of the ventricles appears.
The limbs begin to appear.
The Wolffian body.
Müller's duct.
Ova can be distinguished in the ovary.

Fifth day.

Allantois rapidly increases in size, becomes vascular, and filled with fluid.
First and second circulations together; yelk-sac and allantois both aërating.
Limbs distinguishable into segments.
Cartilaginous endoskeleton.
Anus opened.
Auricular septum.
Liquor amnii appears.

Sixth day.

The visceral clefts closing except the first.
Movements of the chick first observed.
Albumen diminishing; vitellus increasing.

Seventh day.

Amniotic contractions observed.
Primitive circulation replaced by second or allantoic.
Chest walls consolidating.

Eighth to Fourteenth days.

First points of ossification.
Horny beak begins to appear.
Yelk-sac diminishes.
Abdominal wall completed by the eleventh day.
Allantois invests the whole embryo, and its (umbilical) arteries rapidly increase in size.
Feathers growing in their sacs (10th—18th days).

Fifteenth to Twentieth days.

Chick moves from lying crossways to a lengthwise position (14th day).
Umbilical vesicle or yelk-sac withdrawn into the abdomen, and umbilicus closed.
Air chamber at broad end of shell increases.
Chick hatched at end of three weeks' incubation.

35. CHRONOLOGY OF THE HUMAN FŒTUS.

I. month, 1st and 2nd week—Neural groove and notochord.
  Splitting of mesoblast.
  Formation of amnion.
  Appearance of tubular heart.
  Primitive or vitelline circulation.
  3rd week—Protovertebræ.
  Visceral clefts and arches.
  Allantois appears.
  Cerebral vesicles.
  Wolffian body.
  4th week—Limbs show as buds.
  Septum ventriculorum begins.
  Lungs appear as diverticula from the fore-gut.

II. month, 5th week—Aorta formed.
  Duct of Müller.
  Vascular allantois.
  Clavicle and mandible begin to ossify.
  6th week—Visceral clefts disappear.
  Umbilical sac attains its full growth.
  Muscles distinguishable.
  7th week—Germs of teeth appear.
  Ossification of bones of face and limbs.
  8th week—Septum auriculorum begins.
  Lens formed from epiblast.
  Adrenals appear.
  Elbow and knee distinguishable.

III. month—Fœtal placenta begins to form.
  Sex of fœtus distinguishable.
  Fissure of Sylvius appears.

IV. ,, Adipose tissue takes the place of embryonic connective.

V. ,, Hair covers the scalp.

VI. ,, Nails appear.
  Cerebrum grows backwards over cerebellum.

VII. ,, Cerebral convolutions begin to form.

VIII. ,, Ossific points rapidly laid down.

IX. ,, Descent of the testes into the scrotum.

36. GENERAL STATISTICS OF THE HUMAN BODY.

OF ITS PRINCIPAL CONSTITUENTS AND OF THE VISCERA.

Average weight of an adult man, standing 5ft. 8in. and 35 years old, may be taken at 150 pounds, or at 69·5 kilogrammes (nearly 11 stone or 154 lbs.) A man standing 5ft. 6in. should weigh about 10 stone or 140 lbs.; one of 5ft. 7in. 145 lbs.; a short man of 5ft. 1in. should weigh 120 lbs., and a tall one of 6ft., 170 lbs.

Weight of a woman of 30, standing 5ft. 2in., should be about 120 lbs., or 55 kilos.

Weight of new-born child—male, 6—7 lbs., or about 3000 grammes; female, somewhat less. (Note.—The average weight of the still-born fœtus at full time is greater than that of children born alive.)

Weight of child one year old, about 20 lbs., or above 10 kilos.
,,   4 years old, 33·5 — 35 lbs.
,,   10   ,,   50 — 55 ,,
,,   16   ,,   95 — 100 ,,

A man of ten stone, and 5ft. 8in. high, should have a chest girth of somewhat over a yard, 37 or 38 inches. A short man of 5ft. 1in. should have 34in. girth; and a tall one of 6ft., 40 or 41in., *i.e.*, somewhat over a metre.

Water.

Water makes up nearly 90lbs. of the total weight of the body, *i.e.*—about two-thirds altogether: or three-fourths, excluding the bones. In the new-born child it constitutes about 65 per cent.

In the several parts of the body there is present of water :—

In the Vitreous humour	98	per cent.
,, Serum	95	,,
,, Blood, about	80	,,
,, Brain and Muscles, about	75–77	,,
,, Spinal cord	70	,,
,, Liver	70	,,
,, Cartilage and elastic tissue	50	,,
,, Bone	15–20	,,
,, Enamel	0	,,

APPENDIX OF NOTES AND TABLES. 97

Salts.

The mineral Salts pervade all the liquids and tissues, but in small quantities, except in the bones.

In *serum, urine* and the other liquids, sodic chloride is by far the most abundant salt; next, sodic carbonates and phosphates; then, earthy phosphates and alkaline sulphates.

In the *muscles*, blood corpuscles and soft parts generally, potash salts and phosphates are more abundant.

In the *bones*, after removing water and fatty matter, a third by weight consists of animal matter, chiefly collagen, which yields gelatin on boiling : 34 per cent. More than half is bone-earth, $Ca_3 2PO_4$: 51 per cent. About a tenth is chalk, $CaCO_3$: 11 per cent. Calcic Fluoride makes up nearly two per cent. Magnesium phosphate rather more than one per cent., and there are only traces of chlorides and sulphates.

Fatty Constituents.

The amount of Fat varies greatly within the limits of health. More abundant in infancy than in adult life, in women than in men. Usually least so between 10 and 20 in males, between 10 and 16 in females. Most abundant under 5 and over 50.

For a man of 35, weighing 150lbs., about 28lbs. has been given as a normal amount of adipose tissue, *i.e.* about 18 per cent.; for a woman, 25 per cent.; and for a growing lad, about 12 per cent.

In Adipose tissue itself there is 82·5 per cent. of fat.
Yellow marrow ... ... 95 ,,
Brain ... ... 20 ,,
Yelk of egg ... ... 12 ,,
Milk ... ... 4·5 ,,
Hair (from the sebum)... 4 ,,
Muscle ... ... 3—4 ,,
Liver ... ... as much or more ,,
Bone ... ... 1 or less ,,
Blood ... ... ·5 ,,

The several Organs.

Of the 150lbs. weight of the body—

The SKELETON weighs ... ... 25lbs., or about 16 p. c.
MUSCLES (with tendons and fasciæ) 65—70lbs. or nearly half.
ADIPOSE TISSUE ... ... 25—30lbs. or 15—20 p. c.
SKIN, HAIR, &c. ... ... 10lbs.

The BLOOD which runs off during an autopsy is not more than five or six pints; but probably nearly as much remains in the tissues. The total amount of blood in the body has been reckoned at 12lbs., or nearly a twelfth.

The entire BRAIN in *men* most often weighs between 46 and 52 oz. The average weight has been found in 560 male brains to be 48 oz., in another set of 62 to be 49·5 oz., and in a third of 700 to be 47·7 oz.

An adult *woman's* brain usually weighs between 42 and 46 oz. Among 347, the average was found to be 43 oz., and in 760 other examples it was also 43.

The above figures apply to European brains. The average weight of the brain is less in the Negro, and somewhat greater among the Chinese.

The brain of a new-born *child* weighs as much as 10 oz. in a girl, and 11 oz. or more in a boy. At seven years old it has attained very nearly its full size.

The LIVER weighs from 55 to 60 oz. in an adult man; from 45 to 50 in a woman.

The male HEART weighs 10 or 10·5 oz., the female heart 9 to 10 oz.

The two KIDNEYS weigh from 9 to 10 oz.

The PANCREAS weighs about 3 oz., but varies much without being atrophied or diseased.

The SPLEEN varies still more in weight: 6—10 oz. include the most common weights between the age of 20 and 40. After 45, like other lymphatic organs, it wastes.

APPENDIX OF NOTES AND TABLES. 99

37. BRITISH WEIGHTS AND MEASURES.

20 grains = one Scruple.
30 „ = half-a-drachm.
60 „ = one Drachm.
219 „ = half-an-ounce.
437·5 „ = one Ounce (Avoirdupois) of the
British Pharmacopœia.
875 „ = two ounces.
1750 „ = four ounces or a quarter pound.
3500 „ = eight ounces or half-a-pound.
7000 „ = sixteen ounces or one Pound.
10,500 „ = one Pound-and-a-half.
8,750 „ = one Pint of water.
70,000 „ = one Gallon of water.

---

14 pounds = 1 Stone.
112 „ = 8 stone = 1 Cwt.
2240 „ = 20 cwt. = 1 Ton.

---

12 lines ... ... = 1 Inch, *i.e.*, $\frac{1}{39 \cdot 139}$ of a pendulum
beating seconds.
12 inches ... ... = 1 Foot.
36 „ ... ... = 3 feet = one Yard.
1760 yards or 5280 feet = 1 Mile.

½ minim ... = a drop of proof spirit or tincture.
1 „ ... = ·9 grain of water.
1·1 „ ... = 1 drop of water.
1·5 „ ... = 1 drop of castor-oil.
60 „ ... = 1 fluid drachm or small teaspoonful.
3 fluid drachms = 1 small dessertspoonful.
4 „ = 1 small tablespoonful or half-an-ounce.
8 „ = 1 fluid ounce or 437·5 grains of water.

H 2

APPENDIX OF NOTES AND TABLES.

    10 fluid ounces   = half a pint.
    16   ,,   = 1 pound of water.
    20   ,,   = 1 pint = 34·5 cubic in. = 1·25 lb. water.
    40   ,,   = 2 pints = 1 quart.
    160   ,,   = 8 pints = 4 quarts = 1 gallon = 10
                                   lbs. or 70,000 gr. of water.

---

    4 cubic inches of water weigh nearly 1000 grains.
    100   ,,   ,,   ,,   25,000   ,,
    100   ,,   of CO_2 weigh 47, of air 31, and of H only 2 grs.

38. CENTIGRADE WEIGHTS AND MEASURES.

    1 gramme or gram = one c. c. of water at 4° C. (39·2° F.)
    10 grams   ...   = 1 decagramme.
    100 ,,   ...   = 1 hectogramme.
    1000 ,,   ...   = 1 kilogramme.
    $\frac{1}{10}$ of a gram ...   = 1 decigramme.
    $\frac{1}{100}$,,   ...   = 1 centigramme.
    $\frac{1}{1000}$,,   ...   = 1 milligramme.
    1 metre or meter = $\frac{1}{40000000}$ of a great meridian (as
                                    was supposed in 1790).
    1000 meters   ...   = 1 kilometre.
    $\frac{1}{10}$ of a meter ...   = 1 decimetre = 10 centimetres.
    $\frac{1}{100}$,,   ...   = 1 centimetre or 0·01 m.
    $\frac{1}{1000}$,,   ...   = 1 millimetre or 0·001 m.
    $\frac{1}{1000}$ of a millimeter = 1 micromillimeter (μ.)

---

    1 cubic centimeter or millilitre of water weighs 1 gram.
        1000 c. c. = 1 litre = 1 kilogram of water.

39. COMPARISON OF BRITISH AND CENTIGRADE WEIGHTS AND MEASURES.

    0·0154 grain ...   ...   = 1 milligramme.
    1   ,, ...   = 0·0648 gramme or nearly $\frac{1}{15}$
    1·54 grains ...   ...   = 1 decigramme.
    5   ,, ...   = ·324 of a gramme.

APPENDIX OF NOTES AND TABLES. 101

10 grains		= ·648 of a gramme.	
15·432 ,,		= 1 gramme (= nearly 15½ gr.)	
31 ,,		= 2 grammes (nearly).	
60 ,, or 1 drachm		= 3·77 ,,	
120 ,, or 2 drachms		= 7·5 ,,	
180 ,, or 3 ,,		= 11 ,,	
240 gr. or 4 dr. or ½ oz...		= 14· ,,	
8 dr. or 1 oz.		= 28·3495 ,,	
2 oz.		= 56·7 ,,	
3 ,,		= 85· ,,	
1550 grains or 3½ oz.		= 100 gms. or 1 hectogm. (nearly).	
4 oz. or ¼ lb.		= 113·4 ,,	
7 ,,		= 200 or 2 hectogrammes.	
8 ,, or ½ lb.		= 227 grammes (nearly).	
10 ,,		= 283·5 ,,	
12 ,,		= 340 ,,	
14 ,,		= 400 ,,	
16 ,, or 1 lb. or 7000 gr.		= 453·59 ,,	
1½ lb.		= 680 ,,	
2 lbs.		= 907 ,,	
2·2 ,, or 15,500 grs.		= 1000 ,, or 1 kilogramme.	
3 ,,		= 1360 ,,	
4 ,,		= 1814 ,,	
6 ,,		= 2721 ,,	
8 ,,		= 3628 ,,	
11 ,,		= 5000 ,, or 5 kilograms.	
15 ,,		= 6800 ,,	
18 ,,		= 8163 ,,	
22 ,,		= 10 kilograms.	
44 ,,		= 20 ,,	
66 ,,		= 30 ,,	
88 ,,		= 40 ,,	
110 ,,		= 50 ,,	
112 ,, or 1 cwt.		= 51 ,, (nearly).	
154 ,, or 11 stone		= 70 ,, ,,	
20 cwt. or 1 ton		= 1000 ,, ,,	

1 millimeter	=	$\frac{1}{25}$ inch or ·039 in.
2 millimeters	=	1 line (nearly) ·08 in.
5 ,,	=	$\frac{1}{5}$ inch.
1 centimeter	=	$\frac{2}{5}$,,
2·54 centimeters	=	1 ,,
5 ,,	=	2 inches.
1 decimeter	=	3·937 (nearly 4) inches.
30·5 centimeters	=	1 foot.
61 ,,	=	2 feet.
91·5 ,,	=	1 yard.
1 meter	=	39·37079 inches or $\frac{35}{32}$.
,,	=	1·1 yard nearly.
1 decameter	=	11 yards.
1 kilometer	=	1093 ,, = ·62138 mile.
1·609 kilometer	=	1 mile.
8 kilometers	=	5 miles.
40 ,,	=	25 ,,
100 ,,	=	62 ,,
160 ,,	=	100 ,,

1 cubic centimeter or gram of water	=	16 minims.
2 cubic centimeters	=	32 ,,
4 ,,	=	1 fluid drachm (nearly).
7·5 ,,	=	2 ,,
14 ,,	=	4 ,,
28·4 ,,	=	1 fluid ounce.
100 ,,	=	$3\frac{1}{2}$ fluid ounces.
284 ,,	=	10 oz. or $\frac{1}{2}$ pint.
568 ,,	=	1 pint = 34·5 cubic inches.
1000 c. c. or 1 litre	=	1·76 pints.
1136 c. c. or 1·1 litre	=	1 quart.
4544 c. c. or $4\frac{1}{2}$ litres	=	1 gallon or 8 pints or 10 lbs. of water.

To convert the expression for the strength of a solution in terms of grammes to the litre into terms of grains to a pint (approximately), multiply by 9.

40. EQUIVALENT FAHRENHEIT AND CENTIGRADE SCALES.

Fahr.			Cent.
212°	corresponds	with	100°
203°	,,	,,	95°
194°	,,	,,	90°
185°	,,	,,	85°
176°	,,	,,	80°
167°	,,	,,	75°
158°	,,	,,	70°
149°	,,	,,	65°
140°	,,	,,	60°
131°	,,	,,	55°
122°	,,	,,	50°
113°	,,	,,	45°
111·2°	,,	,,	44°
109·4°	,,	,,	43°
107·6°	,,	,,	42°
105·8°	,,	,,	41°
104°	,,	,,	40°
102·2°	,,	,,	39°
100·4°	,,	,,	38°
98·6°	,,	,,	37°
96·8°	,,	,,	36°
95°	,,	,,	35°
86°	,,	,,	30°
77°	,,	,,	25°
68°	,,	,,	20°
59°	,,	,,	15°
50°	,,	,,	10°
41°	,,	,,	5°
32°	,,	,,	0°

5° C. = 9° F.
To turn C. into F. × 9 ÷ 5 + 32.
To turn F. to C. − 32 × 5 ÷ 9.

41. SOME OF THE MORE IMPORTANT NAMES AND DATES IN THE HISTORY OF PHYSIOLOGY, ARRANGED UNDER HEADS.

I. ANATOMY.

ARISTOTELES. Born at Stagira, B.C. 384, died at Chalcis, æt. 62. *De animalibus historia. De partibus animalium. De generatione. De animalium incessu.*
HEROPHILUS. }
ERASISTRATUS. } B.C. 320–260. Alexandria.
CL. GALENUS. A.D. 130–200. Rome. Wrote in Greek.
MONDINI dissected at Bologna, 1315.
VESALIUS. 1514–1564. Fleming. Physician to Charles V. The restorer of Anatomy. Prof. at Padua.
SERVETUS (burnéd 1553). Spaniard. Discovered the pulmonary circulation.
COLUMBUS. *Ob.* 1559. Rome.
FALLOPIUS. *Ob.* 1562. Padua.
EUSTACHIUS. *Ob.* 1574. Rome. *Tabulæ anatomicæ.*
INGRASSIAS. *Ob.* 1580. Naples. Discovered the stapes.
ARANTIUS. *Ob.* 1589. Bologna.
CÆSALPINUS. *Ob.* 1603. Padua.
FABRICIUS ab Aquapendente. 1537–1619. Padua. Discovered valves in veins.
VAROLIUS. 1588. Described the brain.
SPIGELIUS. 1582. Padua. *De hum. corp. fabr.*
RIOLANUS. 1580–1657. Collège de France.
HARVEY. 1578–1657. Proved the muscular structure and active contraction of the heart.
ASELLIUS. *Ob.* 1626. Pavia. Discovered the lacteals, 1622.
BARTHOLINUS (Thomas). 1615–1680. Dane. Discovered the thoracic duct, 1652, in a man.
PECQUET. Dieppe. Discovered the thoracic duct independently, 1651, in a dog.
GLISSON. 1596–1677. *Anatomia Hepatis*, 1659.
BORELLI. 1608–1679. Naples. Muscles and their action.

APPENDIX OF NOTES AND TABLES.   105

WILLIS. 1622–75. *Cerebri Anatome*, 1664.
STENO. 1638–87. Dane. *De Musculis et Glandulis.* 1664.
PEYER. Schaffhausen. *De glandulis intestinorum*, 1665.
HAVERS. *Osteologia nova*, 1691.
BELLINI. 1643–1703. Pisa. *De structura et usu renum*, 1677.
VALSALVA. 1666–1723. Bologna.
ALBINUS. 1697–1770. Leyden. *Historia Musculorum*, 1734.
WINSLOW. *Exposition anat. du corps humain*, 1733.
WM. HUNTER. 1718–1783.
JOHN HUNTER. 1733–1793.
SCARPA. 1747–1832. Pavia. *Anat. Annot.* 1779.
CRUIKSHANK. 1745–1800. *Anatomy of absorbing vessels.* 1786.
SÖMMERING. 1755–1830. Munich. *De corporis humani fabrica.* 1794.
ASTLEY COOPER. 1769–1841. Anatomy of Thymus, of Mamma, of Testis, of Hernia.
GOODSIR. 1814–67. Edinburgh.
CRUVEILHIER. 1789–74. *Traité d' Anatomie descriptive*, 1862.
HENLE. Göttingen. *Handbuch der syst. Anat.* 1855–71.

Textbooks.—Quain's "Anatomy," 9th ed., 2 vols. Ward's "Osteology." Ellis's "Demonstrations of Anatomy." Huxley's "Anatomy of Vertebrated Animals." Flower's "Osteology of Mammalia."

II. HISTOLOGY.

MALPIGHI. 1628–94. Bologna.
LEUUWENHOECK. 1633–1723. Holland. F.R.S.
SWAMMERDAM. 1637–85. Holland.
HOOKE. 1635–1703. Sec. R.S. *Micrographia*, 1667.
GREW. 1628–1711. Curator R.S. *Anatomy of Plants.*

RUYSCH. 1638–1731. Holland. Anatomical Museum of injected preparations.

BICHAT. 1770–1802. Paris. *Anatomie Générale.*

SCHWANN. 1810–82. Liége. Microscopical Researches, 1839.
BOWMAN. On muscle, 1840. On the kidney, 1842.
VIRCHOW. Berlin. *Cellular Pathology*, 1858.

106   APPENDIX OF NOTES AND TABLES.

MAX SCHULTZE. *Ob.* 1873. Bonn.
SHARPEY. *Ob.* 1880, æt. 78. University College.
BEALE. King's College.
RANVIER. Collège de France.

Textbooks.—Sharpey, by Schäfer, in Quain's "Anatomy." Klein's "Elements of Histology." Articles by Max Schultze, Pflüger, Hering, Ludwig, Waldeyer, and Engelmann, in Stricker's "Textbook of Histology" (Sydenham Soc. Transl. 2 vols.)

III. PHYSIOLOGICAL CHEMISTRY.

BOYLE. 1627-1691.
MAYOW. 1645-1679. *De spiritu nitro-aëreo* (oxygen.)
BLACK. 1728-99. Edinburgh.
CAVENDISH. 1731-1810.
SCHEELE. 1742-86. Sweden.
PRIESTLEY. 1733-1804. Birmingham.
LAVOISIER. 1743-1794. Guillotined in the Reign of Terror.

DALTON. 1767-1844. Manchester. Author of the atomic theory.
WOLLASTON. 1766-1828.
DAVY. 1778-1829.
BERZELIUS. 1779-1848. Sweden.
MARCET. 1770-1822.
GAY-LUSSAC. 1778-1850.
PROUT. 1786-1850.
CHEVREUIL. *Nat.* 1786.
WÖHLER. 1802-1882. Göttingen. Made Urea, 1828.
LIEBIG. 1803-73. Giessen, Munich.
DUMAS. 1800-83. Paris.
MULDER. 1803-77. Utrecht.
GRAHAM. 1805-69.
GOLDING BIRD. 1814-1854.
BERTHELOT. *Nat.* 1827. Collège de France.
GERHARDT 1816-56 and LAURENT. 1807-53.
J. F. SIMON. Berlin. Textbook. 1842.
GMELIN. Göttingen. Textbook. 1852.
LEHMANN. Leipzig. Textbook. 1859.
GORUP-BESANEZ. 1817-78. Erlangen. Textbook.

APPENDIX OF NOTES AND TABLES.   107

WURTZ. *Ob.* 1884. Paris.
HOPPE SEYLER. Strassburg. Textbook. 1877.
KÜHNE. Heidelberg. Textbook. 1868.
PARKES. *Ob.* 1876. Netley.
LIEBREICH. Berlin.
PAVY.
GILBERT and LAWES. Rothampstead.

Textbooks.—Gamgee's "Physiological Chemistry of the Animal Body." Lea's Appendix to " Foster's Textbook of Physiology." Charles's "Physiological and Pathological Chemistry."

IV. GENERAL PHYSIOLOGY.

The Physical Apparatus of Digestion, Circulation, Respiration, and Secretion.

HARVEY. 1578–1557. *De Motu Cordis et Sanguinis.* 1628.
MALPIGHI. 1628–94. Bologna. Demonstrated the capillary circulation.
LOWER. 1631–91. *De corde.* 1669.
MAYOW. 1645–79. *De respiratione.* 1673.

HALES. 1677–1761. Rector of Farringdon. *Hœmastatics.* 1733.
HALLER. 1708–1777. Göttingen. *Elementa Physiologiœ.* 1757.
REAUMUR. 1683–1757. Paris. Experiments on Digestion.
JOHN HUNTER. 1728–1793. Treatise on the Blood.
HEWSON. 1739–1774. Experimental inquiry into the properties of the Blood. 1771.
SPALLANZANI. 1729–1799. Naples. Experiments on digestion and respiration.

MAGENDIE. 1783-1855. Collège de France.
BEAUMONT. 1825–83. U.S.A. Observations on St. Martin.

JOHANNES MÜLLER. 1801–1858. Berlin. Treatise on Glands.
E. H. WEBER. *Ob.* 1878. Leipzig.
VOLKMANN. 1801–1877. Monograph on the Circulation.
SCHWANN. 1810–1882. Liége. Digestion, arteries, &c.

108   APPENDIX OF NOTES AND TABLES.

BERNARD. 1813-1878. Collège de France. Glycogen, Vasomotor nerves, Pancreas.
LUDWIG. Leipzig. Kymograph, Chorda Tympani, &c.
BRÜCKE. Vienna. Digestion.
TRAUBE. *Ob.* 1878. Berlin. Circulation.
CZERMAK. *Ob.* 1873. Prag. Laryngoscope.
PFLÜGER. Bonn. Secretion.
FICK. Würzburg. Circulation.
CHAUVEAU. Lyons. Circulation.
MAREY. Collège de France. Spring sphygmograph.
HEIDENHAIN. Breslau. Secretion.

Textbooks.—Foster's "Textbook of Physiology," 4th ed. Hermann's "Textbook of Human Physiology," translated by Gamgee. Yeo's "Manual of Physiology."

V. THE NERVOUS SYSTEM AND THE SENSES.

WILLIS. 1622-75. Brain. Reflex action.

PROCHASKA. 1749-1820. Prague. Reflex action.
YOUNG. 1773-1829. Senses.
BELL. 1774-1842. Nerves.
MAGENDIE. 1783-1855. Collège de France. Nerves.
FLOURENS. 1794-1867. Brain.
MARSHALL HALL. 1790-1857. Reflex action.
JOHANNES MÜLLER. 1801-58. Berlin. Nerves, senses.

DU BOIS-REYMOND. Berlin. Nerves.
BERNARD. Collège de France. Nerves.
WALLER. *Ob.* 1870. Nerves.
BROWN SEQUARD. Paris. Nerves.
DONDERS. Utrecht. Nerves.
HELMHOLTZ. Berlin. Eye and Ear. Ophthalmoscope.
PFLÜGER. Bonn. Nerves.
HERMANN. Zürich. Nerves.
FERRIER. King's College. Brain.
GOLTZ. Strassburg. Brain.

Beside the account of the Nervous System and Senses in Foster's and Hermann's Textbooks, may be mentioned Bern-

APPENDIX OF NOTES AND TABLES. 109

Stein's "Five Senses of Man," Bain's "Senses and Intellect," Hemholtz's "Tonempfindungen," and the articles in Hermann's "Handbuch," vols. ii. and iii.

VI. REPRODUCTION AND DEVELOPMENT.

ARISTOTLE. B.C. 333.

FABRICIUS ab Aquapendente. *De formatione Ovi et Pulli.* 1621. Padua.
HARVEY. *Exercitationes de Generatione Animalium.* 1651.
NEEDHAM. *De formato fœtu.* 1668.
MALPIGHI. *De formatione pulli.* Bologna. 1672.
REDI. *Esperienze intorno alla Generazione degl' Insetti;* refuting spontaneous generation. Florence. 1674.
DE GRAAF. Ovaries and ovisacs. Delft. 1677.
SWAMMERDAM. 1605-1685. Yelk cleavage.
LEUUWENHOECK. Discovered spermatozoa.

VALLISNERI. 1661-1730. *De generatione hominis et animalium.* Venice. 1739.
WOLFF. 1735-94. Königsberg. *Theoria Generationis,* 1759, a hundred years before the publication of the "Origin of Species," by Darwin.
HALLER. Göttingen. Development of the heart of the chick. Opposed Wolff's views.

DÖLLINGER. Würzburg. 1816.
PANDER. Würzburg. 1791-1865. Discovered the three layers of the blastoderm. 1817.
VON BAER. 1792-1876. "Development of man and animals." 1828. Discovered the mammalian ovum in 1827. Königsberg. St. Petersburg.
PRÉVOST and DUMAS (afterwards the chemist). 1824-5. Geneva. Development of Frog.
PURKINJÉ. 1825. Discovered the germinal vesicle.
RUSCONI. 1826. Milan. Development of Frog and of Fishes.

APPENDIX OF NOTES AND TABLES.

RATHKE. 1793–1861. Königsberg. Described the visceral arches. Development of viper, tortoise, and other reptiles. 1839–48.

JOHANNES MÜLLER. 1830. Bonn. Müller's duct, &c.

RUDOLF WAGNER. Leipzig. 1835. Discovered the germinal spot.

WHARTON JONES. 1837. Early changes in mammalian embryo.

BARRY. 1840. Early human ovum.

COSTE. 1834–47. Paris.

REMAK. 1820–1865. Berlin. Histology of embryo.

BISCHOFF. Munich. 1807–1882. Development of rabbit, dog, guinea-pig and roebuck. 1840–1854.

KÖLLIKER. Systematic treatise on development. 1801–80. Würzburg.

HIS. Leipzig.

ED. VAN BENEDEN. Liége.

FOSTER and BALFOUR. Development of Chick. 1874.

BALFOUR. Comparative Embryology. 1881.

Textbook.—Allen Thompson's account of the development of the Fœtus in Quain's "Anatomy."

[CATALOGUE C]

LONDON, October, 1884.

J. & A. CHURCHILL'S

MEDICAL CLASS BOOKS.

ANATOMY.

BRAUNE.—An Atlas of Topographical Anatomy, after Plane Sections of Frozen Bodies. By WILHELM BRAUNE, Professor of Anatomy in the University of Leipzig. Translated by EDWARD BELLAMY, F.R.C.S., and Member of the Board of Examiners; Surgeon to Charing Cross Hospital, and Lecturer on Anatomy in its School. With 34 Photo-lithographic Plates and 46 Woodcuts. Large Imp. 8vo, 40s.

FLOWER.—Diagrams of the Nerves of the Human Body, exhibiting their Origin, Divisions, and Connexions, with their Distribution to the various Regions of the Cutaneous Surface, and to all the Muscles. By WILLIAM H. FLOWER, F.R.C.S., F.R.S. Third Edition, containing 6 Plates. Royal 4to, 12s.

GODLEE.—An Atlas of Human Anatomy: illustrating most of the ordinary Dissections and many not usually practised by the Student. By RICKMAN J. GODLEE, M.S., F.R.C.S., Assistant-Surgeon to University College Hospital, and Senior Demonstrator of Anatomy in University College. With 48 Imp. 4to Coloured Plates, containing 112 Figures, and a Volume of Explanatory Text, with many Engravings. 8vo, £4 14s. 6d.

HEATH.—Practical Anatomy: a Manual of Dissections. By CHRISTOPHER HEATH, F.R.C.S., Holme Professor of Clinical Surgery in University College and Surgeon to the Hospital. Fifth Edition. With 24 Coloured Plates and 269 Engravings. Crown 8vo, 15s.

11, NEW BURLINGTON STREET.

J. & A. Churchill's Medical Class Books.

ANATOMY—*continued.*

HOLDEN.—A Manual of the Dissection of the
Human Body. By LUTHER HOLDEN, F.R.C.S., Consulting-Surgeon to
St. Bartholomew's Hospital. Fifth Edition, by JOHN LANGTON,
F.R.C.S., Surgeon to, and Lecturer on Anatomy at, St. Bartholomew's
Hospital. With Engravings. 8vo. [*Nearly ready.*

By the same Author.

Human Osteology: comprising a Description of the Bones, with Delineations of the Attachments of the
Muscles, the General and Microscopical Structure of Bone
and its Development. Sixth Edition, revised by the Author and
JAMES SHUTER, F.R.C.S., late Assistant-Surgeon to St. Bartholomew's Hospital. With 61 Lithographic Plates and 89 Engravings.
Royal 8vo, 16s.

ALSO,

Landmarks, Medical and Surgical. Third
Edition. 8vo, 3s. 6d.

MORRIS.—The Anatomy of the Joints of Man.
By HENRY MORRIS, M.A., F.R.C.S., Surgeon to, and Lecturer on Anatomy and Practical Surgery at, the Middlesex Hospital. With 44
Plates (19 Coloured) and Engravings. 8vo, 16s.

The Anatomical Remembrancer; or, Complete Pocket Anatomist. Eighth Edition. 32mo, 3s. 6d.

WAGSTAFFE.—The Student's Guide to Human
Osteology. By WM. WARWICK WAGSTAFFE, F.R.C.S., late Assistant-Surgeon to, and Lecturer on Anatomy at, St. Thomas's Hospital.
With 23 Plates and 66 Engravings. Fcap. 8vo, 10s. 6d.

WILSON — BUCHANAN — CLARK. — Wilson's
Anatomist's Vade-Mecum: a System of Human Anatomy. Tenth
Edition, by GEORGE BUCHANAN, Professor of Clinical Surgery in the
University of Glasgow, and HENRY E. CLARK, M.R.C.S., Lecturer on
Anatomy in the Glasgow Royal Infirmary School of Medicine. With
450 Engravings, including 26 Coloured Plates. Crown 8vo, 18s.

11, *NEW BURLINGTON STREET.*

J. & A. Churchill's Medical Class Books.

BOTANY.

BENTLEY.—A Manual of Botany. By Robert
BENTLEY, F.L.S., M.R.C.S., Professor of Botany in King's College and to the Pharmaceutical Society. With 1185 Engravings. Fourth Edition. Crown 8vo, 15s.

By the same Author.

The Student's Guide to Structural,
Morphological, and Physiological Botany. With 660 Engravings. Fcap. 8vo, 7s. 6d.

ALSO,

The Student's Guide to Systematic
Botany, including the Classification of Plants and Descriptive Botany. With 357 Engravings. Fcap. 8vo, 3s. 6d.

BENTLEY AND TRIMEN.—Medicinal Plants:
being descriptions, with original Figures, of the Principal Plants employed in Medicine, and an account of their Properties and Uses. By ROBERT BENTLEY, F.L.S., and HENRY TRIMEN, M.B., F.L.S. In 4 Vols., large 8vo, with 306 Coloured Plates, bound in half morocco. gilt edges, £11 11s.

CHEMISTRY.

BERNAYS.—Notes for Students in Chemistry;
being a Syllabus of Chemistry compiled mainly from the Manuals of Fownes-Watts, Miller, Wurz, and Schorlemmer. By ALBERT J. BERNAYS, Ph.D., Professor of Chemistry at St. Thomas's Hospital. Sixth Edition. Fcap. 8vo, 3s. 6d.

By the same Author.

Skeleton Notes on Analytical Chemistry,
for Students in Medicine. Fcap. 8vo, 2s. 6d.

BLOXAM.—Chemistry, Inorganic and Organic;
with Experiments. By CHARLES L. BLOXAM, Professor of Chemistry in King's College. Fifth Edition. With 292 Engravings. 8vo, 16s.

By the same Author.

Laboratory Teaching; or, Progressive
Exercises in Practical Chemistry. Fourth Edition. With 83 Engravings. Crown 8vo, 5s. 6d.

11, *NEW BURLINGTON STREET.*

J. & A. Churchill's Medical Class Books.

CHEMISTRY—*continued.*

BOWMAN AND BLOXAM.—Practical Chemistry, including Analysis. By JOHN E. BOWMAN, formerly Professor of Practical Chemistry in King's College, and CHARLES L. BLOXAM, Professor of Chemistry in King's College. With 98 Engravings. Seventh Edition. Fcap. 8vo, 6s. 6d.

BROWN. — Practical Chemistry: Analytical Tables and Exercises for Students. By J. CAMPBELL BROWN, D.Sc. Lond., Professor of Chemistry in University College, Liverpool. Second Edition. 8vo, 2s. 6d.

CLOWES.—Practical Chemistry and Qualitative Inorganic Analysis. An Elementary Treatise, specially adapted for use in the Laboratories of Schools and Colleges, and by Beginners. By FRANK CLOWES, D.Sc., Professor of Chemistry in University College, Nottingham. Third Edition. With 47 Engravings. Post 8vo, 7s. 6d.

FOWNES.—Manual of Chemistry.—*See WATTS.*

LUFF.—An Introduction to the Study of Chemistry. Specially designed for Medical and Pharmaceutical Students. By A. P. LUFF, F.I.C., F.C.S., Lecturer on Chemistry in the Central School of Chemistry and Pharmacy. Crown 8vo, 2s. 6d.

TIDY.—A Handbook of Modern Chemistry, Inorganic and Organic. By C. MEYMOTT TIDY, M.B., Professor of Chemistry and Medical Jurisprudence at the London Hospital, 8vo, 16s.

VACHER.—A Primer of Chemistry, including Analysis. By ARTHUR VACHER. 18mo, 1s.

VALENTIN.—Chemical Tables for the Lecture-room and Laboratory. By WILLIAM G. VALENTIN, F.C.S. In Five large Sheets, 5s. 6d.

11, *NEW BURLINGTON STREET.*

J. & A. Churchill's Medical Class Books.

CHEMISTRY—*continued.*

VALENTIN AND HODGKINSON.—A Course of Qualitative Chemical Analysis. By W. G. VALENTIN, F.C.S. Sixth Edition by W. R. HODGKINSON, Ph.D. (Wurzburg), Demonstrator of Practical Chemistry in the Science Training Schools. With Engravings. 8vo, 7s. 6d.

WATTS.—Physical and Inorganic Chemistry. By HENRY WATTS, B.A., F.R.S. (being Vol. I. of the Thirteenth Edition of Fownes' Manual of Chemistry). With 150 Wood Engravings, and Coloured Plate of Spectra. Crown 8vo, 9s.

By the same Author.

Chemistry of Carbon-Compounds, or Organic Chemistry (being Vol. II. of the Twelfth Edition of Fownes' Manual of Chemistry). With Engravings. Crown 8vo, 10s.

CHILDREN, DISEASES OF.

DAY.—A Treatise on the Diseases of Children. For Practitioners and Students. By WILLIAM H. DAY, M.D., Physician to the Samaritan Hospital for Women and Children. Crown 8vo, 12s. 6d.

ELLIS.—A Practical Manual of the Diseases of Children. By EDWARD ELLIS, M.D., late Senior Physician to the Victoria Hospital for Sick Children. With a Formulary. Fourth Edition. Crown 8vo, 10s.

SMITH.—On the Wasting Diseases of Infants and Children. By EUSTACE SMITH, M.D., F.R.C.P., Physician to H.M. the King of the Belgians, and to the East London Hospital for Children. Fourth Edition. Post 8vo, 8s. 6d.

By the same Author.

A Practical Treatise on Disease in Children. 8vo, 22s.

STEINER.—Compendium of Children's Diseases; a Handbook for Practitioners and Students. By JOHANN STEINER, M.D. Translated by LAWSON TAIT, F.R.C.S., Surgeon to the Birmingham Hospital for Women, &c. 8vo, 12s. 6d.

11, *NEW BURLINGTON STREET.*

J. & A. Churchill's Medical Class Books.

DENTISTRY.

***GORGAS.*— Dental Medicine : a Manual of**
Dental Materia Medica and Therapeutics, for Practitioners and Students. By FERDINAND J. S. GORGAS, A.M., M.D., D.D.S., Professor of Dentistry in the University of Maryland; Editor of "Harris's Principles and Practice of Dentistry," &c. Royal 8vo, 14s.

***SEWILL.*—The Student's Guide to Dental**
Anatomy and Surgery. By HENRY E. SEWILL, M.R.C.S., L.D.S., late Dental Surgeon to the West London Hospital. Second Edition. With 78 Engravings. Fcap. 8vo, 5s. 6d.

***STOCKEN.*—Elements of Dental Materia Medica**
and Therapeutics, with Pharmacopœia. By JAMES STOCKEN, L.D.S.R.C.S., late Lecturer on Dental Materia Medica and Therapeutics and Dental Surgeon to the National Dental Hospital; assisted by THOMAS GADDES, L.D.S. Eng. and Edin. Third Edition. Fcap. 8vo, 7s. 6d.

***TAFT.*—A Practical Treatise on Operative**
Dentistry. By JONATHAN TAFT, D.D.S., Professor of Operative Surgery in the Ohio College of Dental Surgery. Third Edition. With 134 Engravings. 8vo, 18s.

***TOMES (C. S.).*—Manual of Dental Anatomy,**
Human and Comparative. By CHARLES S. TOMES, M.A., F.R.S. Second Edition. With 191 Engravings. Crown 8vo, 12s. 6d.

***TOMES (J. and C. S.).*—A Manual of Dental**
Surgery. By JOHN TOMES, M.R.C.S., F.R.S., and CHARLES S. TOMES, M.A., M.R.C.S., F.R.S. ; Lecturer on Anatomy and Physiology at the Dental Hospital of London. Third Edition. With many Engravings, Crown 8vo. [*In the press.*

EAR, DISEASES OF.

***BURNETT.*—The Ear: its Anatomy, Physio-**
logy, and Diseases. A Practical Treatise for the Use of Medical Students and Practitioners. By CHARLES H. BURNETT, M.D., Aural Surgeon to the Presbyterian Hospital, Philadelphia. With 87 Engravings. 8vo, 18s.

***DALBY.*—On Diseases and Injuries of the Ear.**
By WILLIAM B. DALBY, F.R.C.S., Aural Surgeon to, and Lecturer on Aural Surgery at, St. George's Hospital. Second Edition. With Engravings. Fcap. 8vo, 6s. 6d.

11, *NEW BURLINGTON STREET.*

J. & A. Churchill's Medical Class Books.

EAR, DISEASES OF—*continued.*

JONES.—A Practical Treatise on Aural Surgery. By H. MACNAUGHTON JONES, M.D., Professor of the Queen's University in Ireland, late Surgeon to the Cork Ophthalmic and Aural Hospital. Second Edition. With 63 Engravings. Crown 8vo, 8s. 6d.

By the same Author.

Atlas of the Diseases of the Membrana Tympani. In Coloured Plates, containing 59 Figures. With Explanatory Text. Crown 4to, 21s.

FORENSIC MEDICINE.

OGSTON.—Lectures on Medical Jurisprudence. By FRANCIS OGSTON, M.D., late Professor of Medical Jurisprudence and Medical Logic in the University of Aberdeen. Edited by FRANCIS OGSTON, Jun., M.D., late Lecturer on Practical Toxicology in the University of Aberdeen. With 12 Plates. 8vo, 18s.

TAYLOR.—The Principles and Practice of Medical Jurisprudence. By ALFRED S. TAYLOR, M.D., F.R.S. Third Edition, revised by THOMAS STEVENSON, M.D., F.R.C.P., Lecturer on Chemistry and Medical Jurisprudence at Guy's Hospital; Examiner in Chemistry at the Royal College of Physicians; Official Analyst to the Home Office. With 188 Engravings. 2 Vols. 8vo, 31s. 6d.

By the same Author.

A Manual of Medical Jurisprudence. Tenth Edition. With 55 Engravings. Crown 8vo, 14s.

ALSO,

On Poisons, in relation to Medical Jurisprudence and Medicine. Third Edition. With 104 Engravings. Crown 8vo, 16s.

TIDY AND WOODMAN.—A Handy-Book of Forensic Medicine and Toxicology. By C. MEYMOTT TIDY, M.B.; and W. BATHURST WOODMAN, M.D., F.R.C.P. With 8 Lithographic Plates and 116 Wood Engravings. 8vo, 31s. 6d.

11, *NEW BURLINGTON STREET.*

HYGIENE.

PARKES.—A Manual of Practical Hygiene.
By EDMUND A. PARKES, M.D., F.R.S. Sixth Edition by F. DE CHAUMONT, M.D., F.R.S., Professor of Military Hygiene in the Army Medical School. With 9 Plates and 103 Engravings. 8vo, 18s.

WILSON.—A Handbook of Hygiene and Sanitary Science. By GEORGE WILSON, M.A., M.D., F.R.S.E., Medical Officer of Health for Mid Warwickshire. Fifth Edition. With Engravings. Crown 8vo, 10s. 6d.

MATERIA MEDICA AND THERAPEUTICS.

BINZ AND SPARKS.—The Elements of Therapeutics; a Clinical Guide to the Action of Medicines. By C. BINZ, M.D., Professor of Pharmacology in the University of Bonn. Translated and Edited with Additions, in conformity with the British and American Pharmacopœias, by EDWARD I. SPARKS, M.A., M.B., F.R.C.P. Lond. Crown 8vo, 8s. 6d.

OWEN.—A Manual of Materia Medica; incorporating the Author's "Tables of Materia Medica." By ISAMBARD OWEN, M.D., Lecturer on Materia Medica and Therapeutics to St. George's Hospital. Crown 8vo, 6s.

ROYLE AND HARLEY.—A Manual of Materia Medica and Therapeutics. By J. FORBES ROYLE, M.D., F.R.S., and JOHN HARLEY, M.D., F.R.C.P., Physician to, and Joint Lecturer on Clinical Medicine at, St. Thomas's Hospital. Sixth Edition. With 139 Engravings. Crown 8vo, 15s.

THOROWGOOD.—The Student's Guide to Materia Medica and Therapeutics. By JOHN C. THOROWGOOD, M.D., F.R.C.P., Lecturer on Materia Medica at the Middlesex Hospital. Second Edition. With Engravings. Fcap. 8vo, 7s.

WARING.—A Manual of Practical Therapeutics. By EDWARD J. WARING, C.I.E., M.D., F.R.C.P. Third Edition. Fcap. 8vo, 12s. 6d.

11, NEW BURLINGTON STREET.

J. & A. Churchill's Medical Class Books.

MEDICINE.

BARCLAY.—A Manual of Medical Diagnosis.
By A. WHYTE BARCLAY, M.D., F.R.C.P., late Physician to, and Lecturer on Medicine at, St. George's Hospital. Third Edition. Fcap. 8vo, 10s. 6d.

CHARTERIS.—The Student's Guide to the Practice of Medicine. By MATTHEW CHARTERIS, M.D., Professor of Materia Medica, University of Glasgow; Physician to the Royal Infirmary. With Engravings on Copper and Wood. Third Edition. Fcap. 8vo, 7s.

FENWICK.—The Student's Guide to Medical Diagnosis. By SAMUEL FENWICK, M.D., F.R.C.P., Physician to the London Hospital. Fifth Edition. With 111 Engravings. Fcap. 8vo, 7s.

By the same Author.
The Student's Outlines of Medical Treatment. Second Edition. Fcap. 8vo, 7s.

FLINT.—Clinical Medicine: a Systematic Treatise on the Diagnosis and Treatment of Disease. By AUSTIN FLINT, M.D., Professor of the Principles and Practice of Medicine, &c., in Bellevue Hospital Medical College. 8vo, 20s.

HALL.—Synopsis of the Diseases of the Larynx, Lungs, and Heart: comprising Dr. Edwards' Tables on the Examination of the Chest. With Alterations and Additions. By F. DE HAVILLAND HALL, M.D., F.R.C.P., Assistant-Physician to the Westminster Hospital. Royal 8vo, 2s. 6d.

SANSOM.—Manual of the Physical Diagnosis of Diseases of the Heart, including the use of the Sphygmograph and Cardiograph. By A. E. SANSOM, M.D., F.R.C.P., Assistant-Physician to the London Hospital. Third Edition. With 47 Woodcuts. Fcap. 8vo, 7s. 6d.

WARNER.—Student's Guide to Clinical Medicine and Case-Taking. By FRANCIS WARNER, M.D., F.R.C.P., Assistant-Physician to the London Hospital. Second Edition. Fcap. 8vo, 5s.

WEST.—How to Examine the Chest: being a Practical Guide for the Use of Students. By SAMUEL WEST, M.D., M.R.C.P., Physician to the City of London Hospital for Diseases of the Chest, &c. With 42 Engravings. Fcap. 8vo, 5s.

11, *NEW BURLINGTON STREET.*

J. & A. Churchill's Medical Class Books.

MEDICINE—*continued.*

WHITTAKER.—Student's Primer on the Urine.
By J. TRAVIS WHITTAKER, M.D., Clinical Demonstrator at the Royal Infirmary, Glasgow. With Illustrations, and 16 Plates etched on Copper. Post 8vo, 4s. 6d.

MIDWIFERY.

BARNES.—Lectures on Obstetric Operations,
including the Treatment of Hæmorrhage, and forming a Guide to the Management of Difficult Labour. By ROBERT BARNES, M.D., F.R.C.P., Obstetric Physician to, and Lecturer on Diseases of Women, &c., at, St. George's Hospital. Third Edition. With 124 Engravings. 8vo, 18s.

CLAY.—The Complete Handbook of Obstetric
Surgery; or, Short Rules of Practice in every Emergency, from the Simplest to the most formidable Operations connected with the Science of Obstetricy. By CHARLES CLAY, M.D., late Senior Surgeon to, and Lecturer on Midwifery at, St. Mary's Hospital, Manchester. Third Edition. With 91 Engravings. Fcap. 8vo, 6s. 6d.

RAMSBOTHAM.—The Principles and Practice
of Obstetric Medicine and Surgery. By FRANCIS H. RAMSBOTHAM, M.D., formerly Obstetric Physician to the London Hospital. Fifth Edition. With 120 Plates, forming one thick handsome volume. 8vo, 22s.

REYNOLDS. — Notes on Midwifery: specially
designed to assist the Student in preparing for Examination. By J. J. REYNOLDS, L.R.C.P., M.R.C.S. Fcap. 8vo, 4s.

ROBERTS.—The Student's Guide to the Practice
of Midwifery. By D. LLOYD ROBERTS, M.D., F.R.C.P., Physician to St. Mary's Hospital, Manchester. Third Edition. With 2 Coloured Plates and 127 Engravings. Fcap. 8vo, 7s. 6d.

SCHROEDER.—A Manual of Midwifery; includ-
ing the Pathology of Pregnancy and the Puerperal State. By KARL SCHROEDER, M.D., Professor of Midwifery in the University of Erlangen. Translated by CHARLES H. CARTER, M.D. With Engravings. 8vo, 12s. 6d.

SWAYNE.—Obstetric Aphorisms for the Use of
Students commencing Midwifery Practice. By JOSEPH G. SWAYNE, M.D., Lecturer on Midwifery at the Bristol School of Medicine. Eighth Edition. With Engravings. Fcap. 8vo, 3s. 6d.

11, *NEW BURLINGTON STREET.*

J. & A. Churchill's Medical Class Books.

MICROSCOPY.

CARPENTER.—The Microscope and its Revelations. By WILLIAM B. CARPENTER, C.B., M.D., F.R.S. Sixth Edition. With 26 Plates, a Coloured Frontispiece, and more than 500 Engravings. Crown 8vo, 16s.

MARSH. — Microscopical Section-Cutting: a Practical Guide to the Preparation and Mounting of Sections for the Microscope, special prominence being given to the subject of Animal Sections. By Dr. SYLVESTER MARSH. Second Edition. With 17 Engravings. Fcap. 8vo, 3s. 6d.

MARTIN.—A Manual of Microscopic Mounting. By JOHN H. MARTIN, Member of the Society of Public Analysis, &c. Second Edition. With several Plates and 144 Engravings. 8vo, 7s. 6d.

OPHTHALMOLOGY.

HIGGENS.—Hints on Ophthalmic Out-Patient Practice. By CHARLES HIGGENS, F.R.C.S., Ophthalmic Surgeon to, and Lecturer on Ophthalmology at, Guy's Hospital. Second Edition. Fcap. 8vo, 3s.

JONES.—A Manual of the Principles and Practice of Ophthalmic Medicine and Surgery. By T. WHARTON JONES, F.R.C.S., F.R.S., late Ophthalmic Surgeon and Professor of Ophthalmology to University College Hospital. Third Edition. With 9 Coloured Plates and 173 Engravings. Fcap. 8vo, 12s. 6d.

NETTLESHIP.—The Student's Guide to Diseases of the Eye. By EDWARD NETTLESHIP, F.R.C.S., Ophthalmic Surgeon to, and Lecturer on Ophthalmic Surgery at, St. Thomas's Hospital. Third Edition. With 157 Engravings, and a Set of Coloured Papers illustrating Colour-blindness. Fcap. 8vo, 7s. 6d.

TOSSWILL.—Diseases and Injuries of the Eye and Eyelids. By LOUIS H. TOSSWILL, B.A., M.B. Cantab., M.R.C.S., Surgeon to the West of England Eye Infirmary, Exeter. Fcap. 8vo, 2s. 6d.

WOLFE.—On Diseases and Injuries of the Eye: a Course of Systematic and Clinical Lectures to Students and Medical Practitioners. By J. R. WOLFE, M.D., F.R.C.S.E., Senior Surgeon to the Glasgow Ophthalmic Institution, Lecturer on Ophthalmic Medicine and Surgery in Anderson's College. With 10 Coloured Plates, and 120 Wood Engravings, 8vo, 21s.

J. & A. Churchill's Medical Class Books.

PATHOLOGY.

JONES AND SIEVEKING.—A Manual of Pathological Anatomy. By C. HANDFIELD JONES, M.B., F.R.S., and EDWARD H. SIEVEKING, M.D., F.R.C.P. Second Edition. Edited, with considerable enlargement, by J. F. PAYNE, M.B., Assistant-Physician and Lecturer on General Pathology at St. Thomas's Hospital. With 195 Engravings. Crown 8vo, 16s.

LANCEREAUX.—Atlas of Pathological Anatomy. By Dr. LANCEREAUX. Translated by W. S. GREENFIELD, M.D., Professor of Pathology in the University of Edinburgh. With 70 Coloured Plates. Imperial 8vo, £5 5s.

VIRCHOW.—Post-Mortem Examinations: a Description and Explanation of the Method of Performing them, with especial reference to Medico-Legal Practice. By Professor RUDOLPH VIRCHOW, Berlin Charité Hospital. Translated by Dr. T. B. SMITH. Second Edition, with 4 Plates. Fcap. 8vo, 3s. 6d.

WILKS AND MOXON.—Lectures on Pathological Anatomy. By SAMUEL WILKS, M.D., F.R.S., Physician to, and late Lecturer on Medicine at, Guy's Hospital; and WALTER MOXON, M.D., F.R.C.P., Physician to, and Lecturer on the Practice of Medicine at, Guy's Hospital. Second Edition. With 7 Steel Plates. 8vo, 18s.

PSYCHOLOGY.

BUCKNILL AND TUKE.—A Manual of Psychological Medicine: containing the Lunacy Laws, Nosology, Ætiology, Statistics, Description, Diagnosis, Pathology, and Treatment of Insanity, with an Appendix of Cases. By JOHN C. BUCKNILL, M.D., F.R.S., and D. HACK TUKE, M.D., F.R.C.P. Fourth Edition, with 12 Plates (30 Figures). 8vo, 25s.

CLOUSTON.—Clinical Lectures on Mental Diseases. By THOMAS S. CLOUSTON, M.D., and F.R.C.P. Edin.; Lecturer on Mental Diseases in the University of Edinburgh. With 8 Plates (6 Coloured). Crown 8vo, 12s. 6d.

MANN.—A Manual of Psychological Medicine and Allied Nervous Disorders. By EDWARD C. MANN, M.D., Member of the New York Medico-Legal Society. With Plates. 8vo, 24s.

11, *NEW BURLINGTON STREET.*

J. & A. Churchill's Medical Class Books.

PHYSIOLOGY.

CARPENTER.—Principles of Human Physiology. By WILLIAM B. CARPENTER, C.B., M.D., F.R.S. Ninth Edition. Edited by Henry Power, M.B., F.R.C.S. With 3 Steel Plates and 377 Wood Engravings. 8vo, 31s. 6d.

DALTON.—A Treatise on Human Physiology: designed for the use of Students and Practitioners of Medicine. By JOHN C. DALTON, M.D., Professor of Physiology and Hygiene in the College of Physicians and Surgeons, New York. Seventh Edition. With 252 Engravings. Royal 8vo, 20s.

FREY.—The Histology and Histo-Chemistry of Man. A Treatise on the Elements of Composition and Structure of the Human Body. By HEINRICH FREY, Professor of Medicine in Zurich. Translated by ARTHUR E. BARKER, Assistant-Surgeon to the University College Hospital. With 608 Engravings. 8vo, 21s.

SANDERSON.—Handbook for the Physiological Laboratory: containing an Exposition of the fundamental facts of the Science, with explicit Directions for their demonstration. By J. BURDON SANDERSON, M.D., F.R.S.; E. KLEIN, M.D., F.R.S.; MICHAEL FOSTER, M.D., F.R.S.; and T. LAUDER BRUNTON, M.D., F.R.S. 2 Vols., with 123 Plates. 8vo, 24s.

YEO.—A Manual of Physiology for the Use of Junior Students of Medicine. By GERALD F. YEO, M.D., F.R.C.S., Professor of Physiology in King's College, London. With 301 Engravings. Crown 8vo, 14s.

SURGERY.

BELLAMY.—The Student's Guide to Surgical Anatomy; a Description of the more important Surgical Regions o the Human Body, and an Introduction to Operative Surgery. By EDWARD BELLAMY, F.R.C.S., and Member of the Board of Examiners; Surgeon to, and Lecturer on Anatomy at, Charing Cross Hospital. Second Edition. With 76 Engravings. Fcap. 8vo, 7s.

BRYANT.—A Manual for the Practice of Surgery. By THOMAS BRYANT, F.R.C.S., Surgeon to, and Lecturer on Surgery at, Guy's Hospital. Fourth Edition. With about 750 Illustrations (many being coloured), and including 6 Chromo-Lithographic Plates. 2 Vols. Crown 8vo, 32s.

11, *NEW BURLINGTON STREET.*

J. & A. Churchill's Medical Class Books.

SURGERY—continued.

CLARK AND WAGSTAFFE. — Outlines of
Surgery and Surgical Pathology. By F. LE GROS CLARK, F.R.C.S., F.R.S., Consulting Surgeon to St. Thomas's Hospital. Second Edition. Revised and expanded by the Author, assisted by W. W. WAGSTAFFE, F.R.C.S., Assistant Surgeon to St. Thomas's Hospital. 8vo, 10s. 6d.

DRUITT.—The Surgeon's Vade-Mecum; a
Manual of Modern Surgery. By ROBERT DRUITT, F.R.C.S. Eleventh Edition. With 369 Engravings. Fcap. 8vo, 14s.

FERGUSSON.—A System of Practical Surgery.
By Sir WILLIAM FERGUSSON, Bart., F.R.C.S., F.R.S., late Surgeon and Professor of Clinical Surgery to King's College Hospital. With 463 Engravings. Fifth Edition. 8vo, 21s.

HEATH.—A Manual of Minor Surgery and
Bandaging, for the use of House-Surgeons, Dressers, and Junior Practitioners. By CHRISTOPHER HEATH, F.R.C.S., Holme Professor of Clinical Surgery in University College and Surgeon to the Hospital. Seventh Edition. With 129 Engravings. Fcap. 8vo, 6s.

By the same Author.

A Course of Operative Surgery: with
Twenty Plates (containing many figures) drawn from Nature by M. LÉVEILLÉ, and Coloured. Second Edition. Large 8vo, 30s.

ALSO,

The Student's Guide to Surgical Diag-
nosis. Second Edition. Fcap. 8vo, 6s. 6d.

MAUNDER.—Operative Surgery. By Charles
F. MAUNDER, F.R.C.S., late Surgeon to, and Lecturer on Surgery at, the London Hospital. Second Edition. With 164 Engravings. Post 8vo, 6s.

SOUTHAM.—Regional Surgery: including Sur-
gical Diagnosis. A Manual for the use of Students. BY FREDERICK A. SOUTHAM, M.A., M.B. Oxon, F.R.C.S., Assistant-Surgeon to the Royal Infirmary, and Assistant-Lecturer on Surgery in the Owen's College School of Medicine, Manchester.
Part I. The Head and Neck. Crown 8vo, 6s. 6d.
  „ II. The Upper Extremity and Thorax. Crown 8vo, 7s. 6d.

11, *NEW BURLINGTON STREET.*

J. & A. Churchill's Medical Class Books.

TERMINOLOGY.

DUNGLISON.—**Medical Lexicon : a Dictionary**
of Medical Science, containing a concise Explanation of its various Subjects and Terms, with Accentuation, Etymology, Synonyms, &c. By ROBERT DUNGLISON, M.D. New Edition, thoroughly revised by RICHARD J. DUNGLISON, M.D. Royal 8vo, 28s.

MAYNE.—**A Medical Vocabulary : being an**
Explanation of all Terms and Phrases used in the various Departments of Medical Science and Practice, giving their Derivation, Meaning, Application, and Pronunciation. By ROBERT G. MAYNE, M.D., LL.D., and JOHN MAYNE, M.D., L.R.C.S.E. Fifth Edition. Crown 8vo, 10s. 6d.

WOMEN, DISEASES OF.

BARNES.—**A Clinical History of the Medical**
and Surgical Diseases of Women. By ROBERT BARNES, M.D., F.R.C.P., Obstetric Physician to, and Lecturer on Diseases of Women, &c., at, St. George's Hospital. Second Edition. With 181 Engravings. 8vo, 28s.

COURTY.—**Practical Treatise on Diseases of**
the Uterus, Ovaries, and Fallopian Tubes. By Professor COURTY, Montpellier. Translated from the Third Edition by his Pupil, AGNES M'LAREN, M.D., M.K.Q.C.P. With Preface by Dr. MATTHEWS DUNCAN. With 424 Engravings. 8vo, 24s.

DUNCAN.—**Clinical Lectures on the Diseases**
of Women. By J. MATTHEWS DUNCAN, M.D., F.R.C.P., F.R.S.E., Obstetric Physician to St. Bartholomew's Hospital. Second Edition, with Appendices. 8vo, 14s.

EMMET. — **The Principles and Practice of**
Gynæcology. By THOMAS ADDIS EMMET, M.D., Surgeon to the Woman's Hospital of the State of New York. With 130 Engravings. Royal 8vo, 24s.

GALABIN.—**The Student's Guide to the Dis-**
eases of Women. By ALFRED L. GALABIN, M.D., F.R.C.P., Obstetric Physician to, and Lecturer on Obstetric Medicine at, Guy's Hospital. Third Edition. With 78 Engravings. Fcap. 8vo, 7s. 6d.

11, NEW BURLINGTON STREET.

J. & A. Churchill's Medical Class Books.

WOMEN, DISEASES OF—*continued.*

REYNOLDS.—Notes on Diseases of Women.
Specially designed to assist the Student in preparing for Examination. By J. J. REYNOLDS, L.R.C.P., M.R.C.S. Second Edition. Fcap. 8vo, 2s. 6d.

SAVAGE.—The Surgery of the Female Pelvic
Organs. By HENRY SAVAGE, M.D., Lond., F.R.C.S., one of the Consulting Medical Officers of the Samaritan Hospital for Women. Fifth Edition, with 17 Lithographic Plates (15 Coloured), and 52 Woodcuts. Royal 4to, 35s.

SMITH.—Practical Gynæcology : a Handbook
of the Diseases of Women. By HEYWOOD SMITH, M.D., Physician to the Hospital for Women and to the British Lying-in Hospital. With Engravings. Second Edition. Crown 8vo. [*In preparation.*

WEST AND DUNCAN.—Lectures on the Diseases of Women. By CHARLES WEST, M.D., F.R.C.P.° Fourth Edition. Revised and in part re-written by the Author, with numerous additions by J. MATTHEWS DUNCAN, M.D., F.R.C.P., F.R.S.E., Obstetric Physician to St. Bartholomew's Hospital. 8vo, 16s.

ZOOLOGY.

CHAUVEAU AND FLEMING.—The Comparative Anatomy of the Domesticated Animals. By A. CHAUVEAU, Professor at the Lyons Veterinary School ; and GEORGE FLEMING Veterinary Surgeon, Royal Engineers. With 450 Engravings. 8vo, 31s. 6d.

HUXLEY.—Manual of the Anatomy of Invertebrated Animals. By THOMAS H. HUXLEY, LL.D., F.R.S. With 156 Engravings. Post 8vo, 16s.

By the same Author.

Manual of the Anatomy of Vertebrated
Animals. With 110 Engravings. Post 8vo, 12s.

WILSON.—The Student's Guide to Zoology :
a Manual of the Principles of Zoological Science. By ANDREW WILSON, Lecturer on Natural History, Edinburgh. With Engravings. Fcap. 8vo, 6s. 6d.

11, NEW BURLINGTON STREET.

www.ingramcontent.com/pod-product-compliance
Lightning Source LLC
Chambersburg PA
CBHW030304170426
43202CB00009B/865